THE
POCKET
SPINE

THE
POCKET
SPINE

Second Edition

Camden Whitaker, MD
Associate Professor, Department of Orthopaedics,
University of Kansas, Wichita;
Orthopaedics and Sports Medicine at Cypress,
Wichita, Kansas

Stephen H. Hochschuler, MD
Chairman and Co-Founder, Texas Back Institute,
Plano, Texas

CRC Press
Taylor & Francis Group
Boca Raton London New York

CRC Press is an imprint of the
Taylor & Francis Group, an **informa** business

CRC Press
Taylor & Francis Group
6000 Broken Sound Parkway NW, Suite 300
Boca Raton, FL 33487-2742

© 2014 by Taylor & Francis Group, LLC
CRC Press is an imprint of Taylor & Francis Group, an Informa business

No claim to original U.S. Government works

Printed on acid-free paper
Version Date: 20140508

International Standard Book Number-13: 978-1-4822-5399-3 (Paperback)

Library of Congress Cataloging-in-Publication Data

Whitaker, Camden, author.
    The Pocket spine / Camden Whitaker, Stephen H. Hochschuler. -- Second edition.
       p. ; cm.
    Includes bibliographical references and index.
    ISBN 978-1-4822-5399-3 (softcover : alk. paper)
    I. Hochschuler, Stephen, author. II. Title.
    [DNLM: 1. Spine--Handbooks. 2. Spinal Diseases--Handbooks. 3. Spinal Injuries--Handbooks. WE 39]

RD768
616.7'3--dc23   2014016706

Visit the Taylor & Francis Web site at
http://www.taylorandfrancis.com

and the CRC Press Web site at
http://www.crcpress.com

Throughout the marathon of my medical training,
there have been few constants.
The one most important and dedicated to me has been my wife,
whose love and understanding have allowed me to complete my training.
To her I owe so much, for which words are inadequate.
Thank you, Heather.

C.W.

Contributors

Rob D. Dickerman, DO, PhD
Adjunct Professor, University of North Texas Health Science Center, Fort Worth; Director of Neurosurgery, Texas Health Presbyterian Hospital Plano; Director of Neurosurgery Spine, The Medical Center of Plano, Plano, Texas

Stephen H. Hochschuler, MD
Chairman and Co-Founder, Texas Back Institute, Plano, Texas

Eduardo Martinez-del-Campo, MD
Postdoctoral Fellow, Biomechanics of the Spine, Division of Neurological Surgery, Barrow Neurological Institute, Phoenix, Arizona

Donna D. Ohnmeiss, DrMed
Texas Back Institute Research Foundation, Plano, Texas

Ralph F. Rashbaum, MD
Co-Founder, Texas Back Institute, Plano, Texas

Hector Soriano-Baron, MD
Postdoctoral Fellow, Biomechanics of the Spine, Division of Neurological Surgery, Barrow Neurological Institute, Phoenix, Arizona

Ryan M. Stuckey, MD

Clinical Instructor, Department of Orthopaedics,
University of Kansas, Wichita; Orthopaedics and Sports Medicine
at Cypress, Wichita, Kansas

Nicholas Theodore, MD, FAANS, FACS

Professor of Neurological Surgery; Chief, Spine Section;
Director, Neurotrauma Program, Division of Neurological Surgery,
Barrow Neurological Institute, Phoenix, Arizona

Camden Whitaker, MD

Associate Professor, Department of Orthopaedics,
University of Kansas, Wichita; Orthopaedics and Sports Medicine
at Cypress, Wichita, Kansas

Foreword

I wish to congratulate Drs. Whitaker and Hochschuler on this exciting new edition of *The Pocket Spine*. They have retained the nicely compact format and have provided generous amounts of information regarding the presentation, evaluation, and nonoperative and operative treatment of various common spinal conditions. It is divided into twelve chapters that can be referenced quickly, with information that is valuable to trainees as well as young practitioners.

The field of spine medicine has grown tremendously over the last decade, and sometimes lost in this explosion of new technologies has been the fact that the majority of conditions that are evaluated and treated by spine physicians have remained relatively constant. Thus it is not unusual for trainees in orthopedic surgery and/or neurosurgical residency and fellowship programs to have difficulty mastering basic concepts and information while concentrating on higher levels of sophisticated diagnostic and surgical interventions. This concise but well-illustrated textbook will provide immediate access to important basic and even somewhat advanced concepts for quick and repetitive learning. In this respect, this book fills an important need in the exploding field of spine technologies.

Highlights of the textbook include outstanding classic illustrations, as well as charts and tables for reference to important data fields. This is especially evident in the early chapters on medical management and head and spine trauma. A chapter on the pediatric spine is worth noting for its thorough description of pediatric spinal deformities in an understandable level.

Again, I commend Drs. Whitaker and Hochschuler and the colleagues who contributed to this new edition on their contribution to spine literature. It will surely continue to be a standard in the laboratory coat pockets of a multitude of medical students, residents, fellows, young practitioners, and other spinal allied health professionals.

Lawrence G. Lenke, MD

Jerome J. Gilden Distinguished Professor and Chief of Spine Service
Washington University School of Medicine
St. Louis, Missouri

Preface

It is hard to believe that 8 years have passed since the publication of the first edition of *The Pocket Spine*. Throughout my training I found certain information extremely important, but I often noticed that studies and information were being misquoted or were difficult to remember. I began keeping note cards in my pocket for ready reference. When those note cards became an unwieldy stack, I began to think of the value to other residents of turning these notes into a book. "Quick reference" was the key—and thus *The Pocket Spine* was born.

The compilation of this book was influenced by the tremendous opportunities I had with orthopedic mentors. In medical school my orthopedic and spine training began with Dr. Marc Asher, with whom I worked, researched, and published. During my residency and further training at the University of Kansas, Wichita, I gained a variety of insights into the art and science of orthopedics by working with thirty staff orthopedic surgeons. As my focus on orthopedics began to narrow to spine surgery, so did the focus of *The Pocket Spine*. During my fourth year of residency, I spent 6 months at the Shriners Children's Hospital in St. Louis, during which I trained with Drs. Lawrence Lenke and Keith Bridwell. From this experience I gathered information on scoliosis. In Plano, Texas, I further refined the book's content during my spine fellowship at the Texas Back Institute. Again with a diverse teaching staff, I benefited from the expertise of eleven spine surgeons, compiling notes on their techniques and sage advice.

Next I spent 6 weeks with Drs. Hillebrand, Albert, and Vacarro and their fellows, focusing on cervical surgery and spine trauma, guided by their experience and depth of knowledge.

This book is intended as a quick and convenient reminder of information for orthopedic residents and fellows, neurosurgical residents, medical students, family physicians, and emergency room physicians. This compact manual covers the spectrum of spinal conditions encountered in the clinical setting. The presentation throughout focuses on clearly delineating the essential points rather than on lengthy narrative. It is my sincere hope that *The Pocket Spine* will prove an invaluable aid to the reader.

Acknowledgment

To all of my mentors I owe great thanks for allowing me into the orthopedic field and then training me in the fascinating complexities of spine surgery. This book is a significant contribution to the spine community that was initiated through the Texas Back Institute Research Foundation's Spine Surgery Fellowship program. I would also like to thank Michelle Berger and the entire Quality Medical Publishing team for their guidance and skill in bringing this book to publication.

Camden Whitaker, MD

Contents

1 ▪ Medical Management

This chapter outlines some of the preoperative and postoperative medical management tools for patients undergoing spine surgery. Because intraoperative management varies depending on the procedure, a lengthy discussion of intraoperative considerations is not included. However, because of the increased incidence of methicillin-resistant *Staphylococcus aureus* (MRSA), the use of vancomycin intraoperatively is presented.

PREOPERATIVE MANAGEMENT

- If the hemoglobin level is not 10 g/dl, give 2 units of packed red blood cells.
- Give antibiotics 30 minutes before incision.
- Patients under 45 years of age do not need a preoperative ECG.

Fluid Maintenance

- Follow for preoperative and postoperative management:

100 ml/kg/hr	First 10 kg
50 ml/kg/hr	Second 10 kg
25 ml/kg/hr	After 20 kg

Treating Fluid Deficits

- Follow for preoperative and postoperative management
- Half in the first 8 hours, then half in the next 16 hours
- 10% dehydrated = 2000 ml loss

  Deficit % × Total weight = Kilogram deficit
  1000 ml = 1 kg

INTRAOPERATIVE MANAGMENT
Using Vancomycin in Cervical, Thoracic, Lumbar, and Pediatric Spinal Surgery

Surgical site infections are a significant source of morbidity and cost associated with spine surgery.[1] They have been reported to complicate 2% to 13% of spinal fusions.[2-5] Risk factors include diabetes, obesity, tobacco use, previous spinal surgery, long operative time, and high blood loss.[6] Administration of intravenous antibiotics within 60 minutes of incision decreases the risk of infection.[7] Resistant organisms such as MRSA are becoming more common and complicate infection prophylaxis.[8] Intraoperative application of powdered vancomycin is gaining ground in spine surgery.[3] The antibiotic doses range from 0.5 to 2.0 g given alone or mixed in cement.[2] Yet optimization of the doses is still in order.[4]

- Benefits
  - Intraoperative local application of vancomycin powder to the wound edges has been shown to lower the risk of wound infection after posterior thoracolumbar fusion.[9,10]
  - This technique has a low cost, achieves high local antibiotic concentration with MRSA coverage, and leads to minimal systemic antibiotic absorption.[9]
  - In this retrospective review of 171 patients undergoing posterior cervical fusion, the infection rate fell from 10.9% to 2.5% ($p = 0.0384$) after the introduction of vancomycin powder.[11]
  - No complications related to vancomycin powder use in spinal surgery have been reported.[5,9,12]
  - Further studies are needed to optimize dosing, assess long-term safety, and evaluate use in other spinal operations.
- Outcomes
  - To date only one study has reported vancomycin concentrations in drainage fluid after spine surgery: in 2006 Sweet et al[5] began

to use adjunctive local application of vancomycin in a total dose of 2 g equally divided between powder form and mixed in with the bone grafting material in posterior instrumented lumbar and thoracic spine surgeries. They measured vancomycin concentrations over 3 days after surgery in 178 of 991 patients. The mean concentrations were 1457, 462, 271, and 128 μg/ml on days 0, 1, 2, and 3, respectively. Variability between lowest and highest concentrations over 3 postoperative days was 8-fold to 23-fold, yet the lowest observed concentration of 48 μg/ml on day 3 was approximately three times the minimum inhibitory concentration (MIC) of resistant strains of *S. aureus*.[6] Another reason for this high variability may be that the concentrations from surgical drains were not stratified by the type of surgery. Reportedly, concentrations of vancomycin in 80% of serum samples were below the detection limit of 0.6 μg/ml. That is in contrast to the findings of Desmond et al,[7] who reported significant serum vancomycin levels after topical application of 0.5 g to sternotomy wounds. Lazar et al[8] reported that of 36 patients whose sternotomy incision was treated topically with 5 g of powdered vancomycin, all had measurable concentrations of serum vancomycin on day 6. Oakley et al[9] reported that all four of their patients who underwent cardiopulmonary bypass had peak serum concentrations of up to 4.4 μg/ml within the first 3 hours and measurable concentrations up to 48 hours after instillation of 1 g of vancomycin powder.

- On the basis of perioperative surveillance of serum vancomycin levels and creatinine, Gans[12] concluded that the local application of 500 mg of vancomycin powder for antibiotic prophylaxis seems to be safe to use in pediatric patients with spinal deformity who have undergone surgery and weigh more than 25 kg, and that this produces no appreciable systemic affects.

POSTOPERATIVE MANAGEMENT

These measures can be used for different postoperative situations as they arise or as needed with adult patients; see Table 1-1 (pp. 6 and 7) for pediatric management.

Hypertension

- Systolic blood pressure >180 and diastolic blood pressure >100
- Nifedipine (Procardia) 10 mg SL q 2 hr prn
- Labetolol 5 to 10 mg IV q hr prn (requires intensive monitoring in CCU)

SAo$_2$

- Titrate if greater than 90%.

Tachycardia

- Consider pain control.

Wound Care

- Every day or as needed for saturation
- Open/contaminated
  - Dalan's solution: Use at one-quarter strength.
  - Apply wet-to-dry dressings once a day.
  - If >4 days, reculture the wound.

Diarrhea

- Antibiotics can cause diarrhea.
- Check for *Clostridium difficile* toxin, white blood cells in feces, leukocytes.
  - If test results are negative, treat with loperamide (Imodium) or bismuth sulfate.

Dermatitis Secondary to Bed Rest

- Treat with Carrington moisture barrier cream or zinc oxide.

Remove Drains

- If drainage is less than 30 ml, remove drain in 24 hours.

Restraints

- Orders must be rewritten every 24 hours.

Temperature

- If the patient's temperature >101.5° F (38.6° C), follow the *Five Ws* of fever management:
  - Day 1: Wind (observe for signs of pneumonia, atelectasis)
  - Day 2: Water (observe for signs of urinary tract infection)
  - Day 3: Wound (observe for signs of wound infection)
  - Day 4: Wonder drugs (observe reaction to drugs, especially anesthetics)
  - Day 5: Walking (walking can help reduce the potential for deep vein thrombosis and pulmonary embolus)
- Order blood cultures × 2, 30 minutes apart from separate sites.
- Give acetaminophen (Tylenol) 10 gr q 4 hr prn.
- Have patient use incentive spirometer 10 times/hr.
- Encourage coughing and deep breathing.
- Rule out urinary tract infection.
- Check medications and wounds.

Pain Management

- Pills
  - Lortab 5 or 7.5: 1 to 2 tabs PO q 4 hr as needed.
  - Oxycodone (Percocet) 1 to 2 tabs PO q 4-6 hr prn.
  - Lorcet 10 is the strongest.
  - Darvocet N 100 causes less nausea.
  - Acetaminophen (Tylenol) 10 gr 1-2 PO q 4 hr prn PO/PR.
- Patient-controlled analgesia (PCA)
  - Meperidine hydrochloride (Demerol) 20 to 60 mg IV q hr prn

Table 1-1 Pediatric Management

Dosage by Patient Weight in Pounds (kg)	IV Fluids	Motrin	Tylenol	Tylenol With Codeine (120 mg + 12 mg)/5 ml	Lortab Elixir (7.5 mg + 500 mg)/15 ml
13 (6)	24 ml/hr	60 mg (3 ml)	90 mg	1.25-2.5 ml q 3-4 hr	0.6 mg (1.8 ml) q 6 hr
18 (8)	32	80 (4 ml)	120	1.5-3.5 ml	1.2 (2.4 ml)
22 (10)	40 D5 ⅓ NS	100 (5 ml)	150	2-4 ml	1.5 (3 ml)
26 (12)	44	120 (6 ml)	180	2.5-5 ml	1.8 (3.5 ml)
31 (14)	48	140 (7 ml)	210	2.75-6 ml	2.1 (4.2 ml)
35 (16)	52	160 (8 ml)	240	3.25-6.5 ml	2.4 (4.8 ml)
40 (18)	56	180 (9 ml)	270	3.5-7.5 ml	2.7 (5.4 ml)
44 (20)	60	200 (10 ml)	300	4-8 ml	3.0 (6 ml)
55 (25)	65	250 (12.5 ml)	375	5-10 ml	3.75 (7.5 ml)
66 (30)	70 D5 ½ NS	300 (15 ml)	450	6-12 ml	4.5 (9 ml)
77 (35)	75	350 (17.5 ml)	525	7-15 ml	5.25 (10.5 ml)
88 (40)	80	400 (20 ml)	600	8-16 ml	6 (12 ml)
99 (45)	85	450 (22.5 ml)	675	10-20 ml	7.5 (15 ml)
110 (50)	90	500 (25 ml)	750	12.5-25 ml	9 (18 ml)

	<10 kg:
	  4 ml/kg/hr
	10-20 kg:
	  2 ml/kg/hr
	>20 kg:
	  1 ml/kg/hr
		Max dose:
		  40 mg/kg/day
		20-40 kg:
		  200 mg q 6-8 hr
		>40 kg:
		  400 mg q 5-8 hr
			Toradol
			<50 kg:
			  15 mg IV q 6 hr
			>50 kg:
			  30 mg IV q 6 hr
			  0.5 mg/kg q 6 hr
				Tylenol
				3 tabs q 3-4 hr
				One tab: 30-50 kg
				Two tabs: >60 kg
					Lortab tablets
					2-5 yr (15-30 kg):
					  2.5 tabs q 6 hr
					5-12 yr (30-50 kg):
					  5.0 tabs q 6 hr
					>12 yr (>50 kg):
					  1-2 tabs q 5 hr

NS, Normal saline.

Dosage by Patient Weight in Pounds (kg)	Morphine	Metoclopramide (Reglan)	Ondansetron (Zofran)	Cefazolin (Ancef)	Clindamycin	Diazepam (Valium)
	0.05-0.1 mg/kg IV q 1-2 hr	0.1-0.2 mg/kg IV/PO q 6-8 hr		50-100 mg/kg/QD divided q 8 hr	10 mg/kg IV q 6 hr	Spasm/CP 0.04-0.2 mg/kg PO q 4 hr
13 (6)	0.3-0.6 mg			100-200 mg		
18 (8)	0.4-0.8			125-250		
22 (10)	0.5-1	1-2 mg	<20 kg: 2 mg IV/PO q 8-12 hr	150-300	100 mg	1-2 mg q 4 hr
26 (12)	0.6-1.2			200-400		
31 (14)	0.7-1.4			225-450		
35 (16)	0.8-1.6			250-500		
40 (18)	0.9-1.6			300-600		
44 (20)	1-2 mg	2-4 mg	20-40 kg: 4 mg	325-650	200 mg	2-4 mg
55 (25)	1.25-2.5			400-800		
66 (30)	1.5-3	3-6 mg		500 mg-1 g	300 mg	3-6 mg
77 (35)	1.75-3.5			500 mg-1 g		
88 (40)	2-4 mg	4-8 mg	>40 kg: 8 mg	500 mg-1 g	400 mg	4-8 mg
99 (45)	2.25-4.5			500 mg-1 g		
110 (50)	2.5-5	5-10 mg		500 mg-1 g	500 mg	5-10 mg
	Demerol 1-1.5 mg/kg IV/IM q 3-4 hr			Gentamicin 2-2.5 mg/kg IV q 8 hr	5 mg/kg PO q 6 hr	Reversal of sedation agent: Flumazenil 10-30 µg/kg IV (200 µg max); >20 kg give 200 mcp

Fentanyl 1-3 µg/kg IV q 2-4 hr
Narcan <20 kg: 2 mg IV, >20 kg: 1 mg/kg

‣ PCA 60 mg loading dose, 10 mg dose, 10-min intervals, 240 mg q 4 hr lockout
- Morphine 2 to 6 mg IV q hr prn
  ‣ PCA 6 mg loading dose, 1 mg dose, 10-min intervals, 24 mg q 4 hr lockout

Nausea

- Metoclopramide (Reglan) 10 mg IV q 6 hr prn
- Prochlorperazine (Compazine) 25 mg PR q 6 hr as needed
- Phenergan 12.5 to 25 mg IV or IM
- Ondansetron (Zofran) 4 mg IV q 4 hr as needed

Sleeping Aids

- Triazolam (Halcion) 0.125 mg HS prn

Laxatives

- X-prep, 1 can
- Milk of Magnesia 30 ml
- Fleet Phospho-Soda 30 ml in 8 oz of water
- Dulcolax PR

Diuretics

- Foley flush (want 0.5 ml/kg/hr)
- Furosemide (Lasix) 20 to 60 mg IV (check potassium level)
- Bumetanide (Bumex) 2 to 4 mg IV
- Hespan (6% hetasback) 250 ml IV over 2 hr

Insulin Sliding Scale: Finger-Stick Blood Sample

151-180 mg/ml	Give 4 U reg SQ × 1
181-220 mg/ml	Give 6 U reg SQ × 1
221-260 mg/ml	Give 8 U reg SQ × 1
261-300 mg/ml	Give 10 U reg SQ × 1
>300 mg/ml	Call

- Hypoglycemia
  - Blood sugar: 40 to 60 mg/ml
    - ▸ Treat with orange juice.
  - Recheck blood sugar if patient becomes symptomatic (shakes)
    - ▸ Treat with ½ amp D50.
- Hyperglycemia
  - As indicated by insulin AccuCheck >300
  - Treat with regular insulin if initial insulin use is:

Minimal	4-6 U
Moderate	10-15 U
Severe	20 U

NG Tube Prophylaxis for Stress Gastritis

- Famotidine (Pepcid) 20 mg IV q 12 hr
- Ranitidine (Zantac) 50 mg IV q 8 hr
- Carafate 1 g PO qid (slurry via NG tube)

Heparin: Anticoagulation

- DVT/PE 80 U/kg bolus, 20 U/kg/hr drip
- Cardiac/other 70 U/kg bolus, 15 U/kg/hr drip
- Adjust for goal aPTT >46 sec for first 16 hr, then 46-70 sec

<37 sec	Bolus 50 U/kg, +4 U/kg/hr, next PTT 8 hr
37-42 sec	Bolus 25 U/kg, +4 U/kg/hr, PTT 8 hr
42-46 sec	No bolus, +2 U/kg/hr, PTT at 8 hr
46-70 sec	Check next AM
70-80 sec	−1 U/kg/hr, PTT at 8 hr
80-115 sec	−2 U/kg/hr at 8 hr
>115 sec	−3 U/kg/hr, PTT at 8 hr; stop infusion in 60 min
>150 sec	Call physician

Warfarin (Coumadin): Anticoagulation

- Coumadin sliding scale

INR	Coumadin (mg)
<1.2-1.3	5
1.4-1.5	4
1.6-1.7	3
1.8-1.9	2
2-3	Hold
3.1-4.0	Hold, 2.5 mg vitamin K PO
4.1-5.9	Hold, 5.0 mg vitamin K PO
>6.0	Hold, 10 mg vitamin K PO

- Reversing anticoagulation

PT >30	Treat with vitamin K SQ
PT >50	Treat with 2 U FFP

Deep Vein Thrombosis Prophylaxis

Medical comorbidities requiring vigilance in the surveillance for deep vein thrombosis (DVT) include a history of CHF, MI, CVA, hypercoagulable states, tobacco consumption, and obesity.[13] The use of TEDS hose and sequential compression devices is sufficient for DVT prophylaxis in the surgical management of the spine.[13] The potential complications of epidural hematoma and subsequent neurologic deterioration and increased need for postoperative blood transfusion are used frequently as arguments against chemical DVT prophylaxis in spine surgery.[13]

- Plexipulse boots, SCD
- Heparin 5000 U SQ q 12 hr (if elevated, then q 8 hr)
- Enoxaparin sodium (Lovenox) 15 mg bid; if a clot occurs, give 1 mg/kg
- D/C Lovenox if PT >14.0

Thromboembolic Prophylaxis for Total Knee Arthroplasty

- Proximal versus distal: Level of trifurcation.
- 2% to 3% clot rate status post venogram.
- Postoperative risks return to preoperative risks at 2 weeks.
- Distal clot: 23% rate of propagation to proximal clot.[13]
- Most clots have occurred by 7 days postoperatively and 80% are detectable.[13]
- Immediately after surgery.

STANDARD POSTOPERATIVE ORDERS

The physician's orders listed in Box 1-1 (pp. 12-14) apply to all patients.

DISCHARGE SUMMARY

The following points should always be included in discharge summaries.

- Admission and discharge date
- Operations/procedures
- Consultants
- Physical examination
- Laboratory tests and radiographs
- Hospital course
- Condition
- Follow-up: Medication, diet, activity, and follow-up appointment

Box 1-1   Physician's Standard Postoperative Orders

Diet
____ NPO
____ NPO/ice chips
____ Regular
____ Clear liquids
____ Advance as tolerated

Laboratory Tests
____ Blood cultures × 2 for temperature >102° F (38.9° C) or shaking chills

Vital Signs
____ Routine recovery room
____ Every 4 hr × 24 hr, then every shift
____ Neurologic check q hr × 8 hr, then every shift (motor, sensory, pulses)
____ Per ICU routine
____ Chest radiograph in recovery room

Activities
____ Bed rest
____ Physical therapy/occupational therapy
____ Ambulation
____ Activities/equipment per protocol
____ Bed positioning
____ Elevate head of bed 30 degrees or to comfort
____ Keep bed flat × _____ days

Fluids and Medications
____ D5 ½ NS at _____ ml/hr when tolerating fluid PO
____ Decrease to TKO or heparin lock
____ D/C after last dose of IV antibiotics
____ Levofloxacin 500 mg PO q 24 hr (start P IV antibiotics)
____ Cefazolin (Ancef) 1 g IV q 8 hr × 3 doses
____ Lincocin 600 mg IGM IV q 12 hr × 3 doses
____ Cephalexin (Keflex) 500 mg PO QID (begin after IV antibiotics are discontinued)

Box 1-1   Physician's Standard Postoperative Orders—cont'd

___ Ciprofloxacin 500 mg PO bid (start after IV antibiotics)

___ Propoxyphene napsylate with acetaminophen (Darvocet N 100) 1-2 PO q 3-4 hr prn for pain

___ Tramadol hydrochloride (Ultram) 50 mg PO q 4-6 hr prn for pain

___ Ketorolac tromethamine (Toradol) 30 mg IV q 6 hr prn × 24 hr prn for pain

___ Oxycodone hydrochloride (OxyContin) 20 mg 1-2 tabs q 12 hr prn for pain

___ Acetaminophen and hydrocodone (Vicodin) 1-2 PO q 4-6 hr prn for pain

___ Lortab 7.5 mg 1-2 PO q 4-6 hr prn for pain

___ Hydrocodone (Norco) 10 mg 1-2 PO q 4-6 hr prn for pain

___ Acetaminophen (Tylenol 3) 1-2 PO q 4 hr prn for pain

___ Acetaminophen (Tylenol) 1-2 PO q 3-4 hr PM H/A and mild pain and fever >101° F (38.3° C)

___ Cyclobenzaprine (Flexeril) 5-10 mg 1 PO tid prn for spasms

___ Diazepam (Valium) 10 mg IM or PO tid prn for spasms

___ Ranitidine (Zantac) 150 mg 1 PO bid

___ Ranitidine (Zantac) 50 mg IV q 12 hr; D/C when taking PO meds

___ Dexamethasone (Decadron) 10 mg IV q 8 hr × 3

___ Morphine PCA

    ___ 1-2 mg q 8-10 min prn with

    ___ 2-4 mg bolus 2-4 hr prn

    ___ 0 mg loading dose

    ___ 30 mg per 4 hr lockout

___ Metoclopramide (Reglan) 10 mg IV q 6 hr

___ Zolpidem (Ambien) 5 mg PO HS PM; may repeat × 1

___ Antacid of choice

___ Senokot S 2 tabs PO HS PM for constipation

___ Promethazine (Phenergan) 12.5-25 mg IV q 4-6 hr PM (if not effective within 2 hr, discontinue)

___ Ondansetron (Zofran) 4 mg IV q 6-8 hr PM (if Phenergan not effective)

___ Diphenhydramine (Benadryl) 25-50 mg PO or IM q 4 hr prn for itching

___ Laxative of choice

___ Preoperative medications per physician

___ Preoperative medications to be resumed are as follows: _____

_____

Continued

Box 1-1   Physician's Standard Postoperative Orders—cont'd

Respiratory
____ Encourage coughing and deep breathing q 2 hr while awake
____ Incentive spirometry q l hr while awake
____ Intermittent positive pressure breathing (IPPB) with albuterol (Ventolin) 0.3 ml
        NS q 6 hr for _____ days
____ Moist air by face tent with compressed air for _____ days

Orthosis
____ Corset/brace
____ Advantage/thoracolumbosacral orthosis (TLSO) (custom molded)

Genitourinary
____ Foley catheter to gravity drainage
____ Tamsulosin (Flomax) 0.4 mg PO QD until patient voids
____ Urecholine 12.5 mg 1 PO q 6 hr × 3 doses or until patient voids
____ Straight catheter if patient is unable to void in 6 hr; if unable to void again,
        insert Foley and if urine output is 200 ml, leave Foley in

DVT Prophylaxis
____ Bilateral lower extremity compression devices
____ TEDS hose
____ Hot ice machine with setup

Dressings
____ Change the dressing every day starting after POD 2 and prn
____ Keep wound dry; Aquashield for showering
____ Patient may shower with supervision after first dressing change with Aquashield
____ Postoperative dressing pack to room

REFERENCES

1. Dakwar E, Vale FL, Uribe JS. Trajectory of the main sensory and motor branches of the lumbar plexus outside the psoas muscle related to the lateral retroperitoneal transpsoas approach. J Neurosurg Spine 14:290-295, 2011.

2. Kanj WW, Flynn JM, Spiegel DA, et al. Vancomycin prophylaxis of surgical site infection in clean orthopedic surgery. Orthopedics 36:138-146, 2013.

3. Vitale MG, Riedel MD, Glotzbecker MP, et al. Building consensus: Development of a Best Practice Guideline (BPG) for surgical site infection (SSI) prevention in high-risk pediatric spine surgery. J Pediatr Orthop 33:471-478, 2013.

4. Chrastil J, Patel AA. Complications associated with posterior and transforaminal lumbar interbody fusion. J Am Acad Orthop Surg 20:283-291, 2012.

5. Sweet FA, Roh M, Sliva C. Intrawound application of vancomycin for prophylaxis in instrumented thoracolumbar fusions: Efficacy, drug levels, and patient outcomes. Spine 36:2084-2088, 2011.

6. Rybak M, Lomaestro B, Rotschafer JC, et al. Therapeutic monitoring of vancomycin in adult patients: A consensus review of the American Society of Health-System Pharmacists, the Infectious Diseases Society of America, and the Society of Infectious Diseases Pharmacists. Am J Health Syst Pharm 66:82-98, 2009.

7. Desmond J, Lovering A, Harle C, et al. Topical vancomycin applied on closure of the sternotomy wound does not prevent high levels of systemic vancomycin. Eur J Cardiothorac Surg 23:765-770, 2003.

8. Lazar HL, Barlam T, Cabral H. The effect of topical vancomycin applied to sternotomy incisions on postoperative serum vancomycin levels. J Card Surg 26:461-465, 2011.

9. Oakley RE, Nimer KA, Bukhari E. Is the use of topical vancomycin to prevent mediastinitis after cardiac surgery justified? J Thorac Cardiovasc Surg 119:190-191, 2000.

10. Kuris E, Moskowitz A. Postoperative drainage and serum vancomycin levels after topical adjunctive application of vancomycin powder in patient with posterior instrumented spine surgery (in press).

11. Strom R. Decreased risk of wound infection after posterior cervical fusions with routine local application of vancomycin powder. Spine 38:991-994, 2013.

12. Gans I. Adjunctive vancomycin powder in pediatric spine surgery is safe. Spine 38:1703-1707, 2013.

13. Rokito SE, Schwartz MC, Neuwirth MG. Deep vein thrombosis after major reconstructive spinal surgery. Spine 21:853-858; discussion 859, 1996.

2 ▪ Imaging of the Spine

Donna D. Ohnmeiss, Hector Soriano-Baron, Eduardo Martinez-del-Campo, Nicholas Theodore, and Camden Whitaker

Imaging is an essential tool in the evaluation of patients with pain or spinal trauma. A variety of techniques are available; the typical course is to begin with the least invasive or least expensive diagnostic tools and progress as necessary to formulate an effective treatment plan. Although imaging is critical to the care of spine patients, it is imperative to keep this in mind: "Treat the patient, not the x-ray." The downside to diagnostic imaging is the fact that not all observed abnormalities are related to symptomatology. Any imaging must be interpreted in terms of the patient's history and the findings on physical examination to complete the diagnostic picture.

PREOPERATIVE IMAGING
Plain Radiograph

The first line of imaging is plain films. In the cervical and lumbar spine, anteroposterior (AP) (Fig. 2-1) and lateral flexion-extension views are the basic views. (See radiograph considerations in Chapter 4 for more information.) A neutral lateral view may be taken as well. If a pars fracture is suspected, oblique views may be helpful. When reviewing plain films one should look for the following: fracture, variations in the appearance of a vertebral body (Fig. 2-2), which may indicate a congenital abnormality, tumor or infection, collapsed disc space (Fig. 2-3), narrowing of the foramen, spondylolisthesis (Fig. 2-4), pars fracture, shape of the pedicles, and symmetry. The flexion-extension views may provide information about instability (Fig. 2-5).

Fig. 2-1 AP radiograph of the lumbar spine showing straight alignment and symmetry.

Fig. 2-2 Lateral view showing abnormality at the L1 level.

Fig. 2-3 Neutral lateral of the cervical spine showing narrowing of the C5-6 disc space.

Fig. 2-4 **A,** Flexion and **B,** extension radiographs of a patient with spondylolisthesis at L4-5.

Fig. 2-5 **A,** Flexion and **B,** extension views are very helpful in identifying abnormal motion, as seen in the two lowest lumbar levels.

In a previously operated spine, one should look for implant-related problems, such as breakage and/or displacement. In patients with a previous fusion, the bone graft should be examined for incorporation. However, unless a blatant nonunion is identified, one should not depend too heavily on plain films for fusion assessment, since it is not highly reliable.

In patients with spinal deformity such as scoliosis or kyphosis, a long film should be taken that provides a view from the upper cervical region to the femoral heads in both the AP and lateral views. In patients with scoliosis, left- and right-bending films are also important to determine the flexibility of the curve.

There is no general consensus in regard to the ideal indications for obtaining radiographs in patients with back pain. From a clinical standpoint, fewer films are desirable because of the expense and radiation exposure. However, from a medicolegal standpoint and for fear of missing the identification of trauma or tumor as soon as possible, early radiographs may be desirable. The North American Spine Society (NASS) has published some guidelines for determining whether obtaining radiographs is appropriate.[1] They recommend that films not be made in patients with an initial episode of back pain of less than 7 weeks' duration unless there are other circumstances related to the pain episode that may be indicative of a serious underlying problem. Such symptoms may include pain at night or when lying down; a motor or sensory deficit that results in bowel or bladder dysfunction; worsening pain despite adequate treatment; a history suggestive of possible fracture or trauma; social factors such as the patient not being able to provide a reliable history; a need for legal evaluation; or a need to determine whether it is appropriate for the patient to engage in certain activities, such as sports. Patients who have a history of significant spine problems or surgery may require earlier imaging. The views obtained should include at a minimum an AP and a lateral view. Lateral flexion and extension films are very helpful in identifying instability and are often substituted for the neutral lateral view.

Magnetic Resonance Imaging

For most patients, the second imaging mode to be pursued is MRI (Figs. 2-6 through 2-8). This is good for assessment of soft tissue, tumors, and infections. The downside of using MRI is that it has been reported that as many as 76% of subjects without back pain who were age and occupation matched to a back pain population had abnormalities on their MRIs.[2] This reinforces the importance of correlating images to clinical findings.

Fig. 2-6 A, Lateral and **B,** axial MRIs show a very large disc herniation at L5-S1.

Fig. 2-7   A, Lateral and **B,** axial views of a large C5-6 disc herniation (same patient as in Fig. 2-3).

Fig. 2-8   MRI of the same patient as in Fig. 2-4. Note the misshapen foramen and abnormal disc at L4-5 resulting from the patient's spondylolisthesis.

> **Red Flag:** One should be cautious if planning surgery based primarily on MRI because of the high false-positive rate.

In previously operated patients, a gadolinium-enhanced MRI may be useful. Images made before and after administration of gadolinium should be compared to aid in distinguishing scar tissue from recurrent disc herniation.

One of the new developments in MRI scanning is upright imaging. This has the potential advantage of imaging the spine when it is loaded. It may also provide the opportunity to scan the spine in various positions. It has been reported that such loaded dynamic imaging of the cervical spine provided additional information in the majority of patients.[3] However, for cervical and lumbar standing imaging, there is a chance of imaging being compromised as a result of artifact created by patient movement, particularly if the scan requires a relatively long time to image.

NASS's recommendation for MRI scanning suggests waiting approximately 7 weeks if the patient has received appropriate care and his or her symptoms have not improved.[4]

A recent article found that patients who underwent MRI of the lumbar spine before the time frame suggested in the guidelines, which allow early imaging in the presence of red flags, had significantly worse outcomes, including extended recovery time and greater treatment costs of approximately $13,000.[5]

> **Red Flag:** An MRI may be performed earlier if the patient has signs of an acute injury, infection, or tumor, or if the patient's neurologic condition is progressively worsening.

Under any circumstances, patients must be carefully screened before the procedure to make certain that the imaging can be performed safely. The screening should focus on any materials that may be affected or moved by the magnetism required for the scans. It should also be noted whether the patient is unlikely, because of claustrophobia, pain, and so forth, to remain still during the imaging.

A high-intensity zone (HIZ) (Fig. 2-9) is defined as a high-intensity signal located in the posterior anulus that is dissociated from the signal from the nucleus and appears brighter than the nucleus.[6] It has been reported that there is a high correlation to HIZ and symptomatic disc disruption identified by discography.[6,7] However, the significance of the HIZ has been questioned in other studies.[8-10]

Fig. 2-9 An MRI showing disc degeneration at L4-5 and L5-S1 levels, identified by the darkness (caused by dehydration) of these discs compared with the normal discs at the cephalad levels. Also note the high-intensity zone (HIZ) at L4-5.

All patients must be carefully screened before an MRI to eliminate possibly exposing patients with functioning electronic implants, such as pacemakers or nontitanium metallic implants, shrapnel, or other metallic fragments, to potentially serious injury from exposure to the magnetic field required for imaging. In addition, MRI imaging may be more difficult, if not impossible, in patients with spinal cord and internal bone stimulators. Patients who are incapable of remaining still long enough to capture a useful image should not be scanned.

Patient movement can significantly compromise the quality of the images, making them difficult to interpret or leading to misinterpretation.

CT Scans

CT scanning has been somewhat replaced by MRI as an early imaging modality in many patients. However, it remains good for imaging bony pathology. In cases of trauma, it may provide greater detail of fracture. It is also useful in the assessment of patients who have undergone fusion to determine if the bone graft has incorporated into a solid mass or growth into metallic fusion cages (Fig. 2-10). As discussed in sections below, CT is very helpful following contrast-based evaluations such as myelography or discography. In the postfusion patient, CT is the method of choice for evaluating patients for possible pseudarthrosis.

Fig. 2-10 Axial CT scanning is helpful in the assessment of fusion incorporation, such as in this patient in whom threaded metallic cages were packed with bone graft.

In addition to assessing bony structures, CT scans provide information helpful in planning anterior interbody spine surgery, such as the choice of fusion or total disc replacement. CT also permits visualization of calcification in the large vessels passing anterior to the lumbar spine (Fig. 2-11).

Fig. 2-11   In addition to the assessment of bony structures, axial CT views are useful for the assessment of vascular structures, which may be helpful in preoperative planning. In this figure, some calcification of the vessels is seen anterior to the spine.

Myelography

Myelography remains the standard for the assessment of problems such as stenosis. The contrast is very helpful in determining the location of the compression of neural tissues. CT scanning after the myelogram is useful to further delineate the location of the compression. Myelography is used for the following situations:

- Unable to obtain an MRI
- MRI is of substandard quality
- Need bony detail
- In older patients with segmental bony stenosis
- Transitional syndrome in patients with old fusion to check for hardware placement

Discography

Although controversial, discography is a useful procedure when performed and interpreted appropriately. NASS has published a document on discography, including indications for the procedure.[11] Indications for discography include, but are not limited to, evaluation of a disc thought to be related to symptoms; assessment of ongoing pain for which other tests have not identified any correlative abnormalities; determination of whether the disc or discs are painful in a segment where fusion is being considered; assessment of candidates for minimally invasive disc procedures; and evaluation of previously operated symptomatic patients to evaluate a disc in a fused segment that is painful, if there is a painful recurrent disc herniation, or to evaluate the disc adjacent to a previous surgery. Discography provides detailed information on the architecture of the disc (see Fig. 2-10). The critical part of the discogram is the assessment of the patient's pain response during the disc injections. This must be interpreted with respect to the patient's clinical symptoms. If the test produces no pain, or pain that is discordant with presenting symptoms, the test is nondiagnostic, regardless of imaged ruptures.

As with myelography, postinjection CT scanning can provide a great deal of additional information. The axial CT views made with contrast medium provide information about the internal architecture of the disc and the exact location and severity of disc disruption and degeneration.

One potential complication of discography is discitis. Although the incidence of complications is low,[12] *persons performing discography should be meticulous in technique*. Any patient complaining of severe pain or new onset of pain after the procedure should be carefully evaluated for discitis (Fig. 2-12, p. 28).

A review study addressed the accuracy of lumbar discography.[13] The authors found evidence-based literature classified as "fair," supporting that discography performed according to the guidelines of

Fig. 2-12   A, Fluoroscopic view of the discographic injection of contrast into the disc spaces. The needle is seen in the L4-5 disc. In both the lateral image **(A)** and the axial CT/discographic image of L3-4 **(B)**, the disc morphology is normal as the contrast remains in the nucleus as injected. The lateral view shows an abnormal L4-5 disc where the contrast passes posteriorly from the nucleus **(A).** The axial CT/discographic image of L4-5 **(C)** provides further information on the disc architecture with the contrast identifying right-sided lateral disc disruption.

the International Association for the Study of Pain may be beneficial in the diagnosis of pain arising from the intervertebral disc.

Bone Scans/SPECT Scans

Bone scans are sometimes used in the evaluation of patients with back pain. They are typically employed to identify "hot spots" of activity; that is, areas of high metabolic activity. This test may be useful in evaluating patients for tumor, infection, or fractures. It has been suggested that single-photon emission computed tomography (SPECT) may be beneficial in identifying patients with pain arising from the facet joints. However, the role of SPECT in back pain patients has not been well defined.

Special Considerations for Imaging in Trauma Patients

Imaging in the early evaluation of trauma patients deserves special consideration (see Chapter 3 for more information). Incorrect diagnosis or missed injuries could have catastrophic consequences for injured patients. It has been noted that the most common reason for missed spinal injuries is inadequate imaging.[14]

A patient's inability or compromised ability to communicate and cooperate with care providers makes it more difficult to evaluate symptoms. Patients who are unable to undergo adequate neurologic evaluation may require more extensive imaging to investigate possible spinal injuries. General recommendations published in a recent review were to perform, as a first evaluation, cervical lateral, AP, and open mouth views (to assess the uppermost cervical vertebrae and the odontoid).[15] The authors stressed the importance of making certain that the lateral views are true laterals with no rotation, image from the upper cervical spine to T1 level, and visualization of the spinous processes. They cited an earlier report that these three views can identify 99% of injuries.[16] Although many other views of the cervical spine may be made, these should be approached only with specific considerations—as well as with extreme caution if the additional views require movement of the acutely injured patient's spine.

Recommendations for imaging evaluation of the thoracic and lumbar spine were to limit this to patients with confirmed cervical injury, calcaneus fracture caused by a fall, regional tenderness, indications of high-impact trauma injuries in the trunk or pelvic regions, or neurologic deficits in a distribution suggestive of injury in the thoracic or lumbar spine.[15] Appropriate plain radiographs are AP and lateral views.

CT scanning can provide excellent delineation of bony injury. In the case of cervical spine trauma, a recent metaanalysis compared plain radiographs with CT scans for the evaluation of patients at risk of cervical injury resulting from blunt trauma.[17] The authors suggested that CT be the initial screening for patients with cervical spine trauma because of its significantly greater sensitivity compared with radiographs. However, they noted that in patients presenting with less risk of significant cervical injury and who can be evaluated well clinically, initial evaluation with radiographs may be sufficient as a screening. Brandt et al[18] advocated the use of CT as an initial screening in trauma patients because of its high sensitivity. They suggested that getting CT scans routinely, rather than plain radiographs, reduces the trauma patient's time in the radiology area, as well as reducing costs and radiation exposure.

MRI has played a lesser role in the early evaluation of trauma patients. However, it is excellent for evaluating soft tissue injuries and swelling. When a bony injury cannot be identified that correlates with symptoms, MRI may be pursued. However, as with any MRI, patients must be carefully screened for any type of metal implants that may make scanning dangerous to the patient.

INTRAOPERATIVE IMAGING

Spine surgery is a very demanding surgical discipline, allowing little room for error while requiring maximum preparation and concentration. It is crucial to use all resources available to achieve the best results possible. One of the most powerful tools available in the operating room is imaging. During the past 25 years, many technologies have been developed, and as a result, intraoperative imaging has become increasingly important to provide accurate surgical results, avoid unnecessary dissection, get quicker and more precise trajectories, and obtain better outcomes.

The exposure of the surgical field allows only two-dimensional visualization. Therefore it is very important for all surgeons to acquire a deep spatial sense to anticipate in a three-dimensional fashion the exact final position of inserted implants.[19]

Plain radiographs are the first line of intraoperative imaging. As mentioned previously in this chapter, the typical course is to begin with the simplest and least expensive diagnostic tools and progress to more complex or more expensive tools as necessary. In the operating room, wrong-level disc surgery, especially in the thoracic region, is a potential and unfortunately common occurrence. The use of AP and lateral view plain radiographs helps the surgeon identify precisely the level of interest. In contrast, oblique radiographs are difficult to obtain during surgery and do not add much useful information. For spinal screw insertion, the axial plane is the most important view, but it is not obtainable with conventional radiographs during surgery.[20]

Fluoroscopy has been used in spine surgery for many years and provides real-time feedback. The drawback of fluoroscopy is that it provides only two-dimensional information in the setting of complex three-dimensional anatomy. It also delivers high doses of radiation to the surgeon and patient, which may be especially unnecessary in minimally invasive procedures. In some studies, disruption of the pedicle cortex ranges from 21% to 31% with fluoroscopy and decreases to 5.5% when axial CT images are used for localization.[20]

Advancements have been made to develop CT scanning and various multidimensional fluoroscopy systems for use in the operating room (Box 2-1). Initially these were most often used for pedicle screw placement in the thoracic and lumbar spinal regions. Currently their applications have expanded to include the cervical spine and sacroiliac joints. There is enthusiasm about the potential benefit of these imaging technologies to provide more accurate device placement, thus reducing complications such as nerve root injury related to malpositioned spinal implants. The primary disadvantage is the cost of these technologies. Also, there is a learning curve in their use. More research is needed to help determine for which procedures and in which patients these systems are cost-effective.

Box 2-1   Intraoperative CT Scan Use

- Maximize screw diameter and length in the thoracic and lumbar spine
- Revision case of the spine
- Extension of cervical fusions to the thoracic spine
- Deformity cases with small pedicles

The Era of Intraoperative Image-Guided Navigation

The need for intraoperative navigation in spine surgery was born out of the neurosurgical experience with image-guided cranial surgery.

Today image guidance based on frameless stereotactic techniques is widely used in spine surgery to better define anatomic landmarks, localize pathologic lesions, assist in creating novel pathways, and facilitate precise instrumentation placement.[21-23] Spinal navigation provides the surgeon with additional three-dimensional information, enhancing the accuracy of surgical procedures. Although computer-assisted surgery was first introduced in the 1980s for the placement of needles and probes into the brain, it was first used for spine surgery in the 1990s.[24]

The benefits of navigation include increased accuracy, reduced morbidity, reduced radiation exposure for patients and surgeons, and improved patient outcomes. Intraoperative navigation is used to provide real-time feedback on position and instrumentation trajectory based on a medical image (e.g., MR or CT). This feedback is achieved by attaching a reference frame to the patient. These frames are usually attached to the tip of a vertebral spinous process. Optical systems with infrared lights are the most commonly used.[24] The reference frame position is triangulated between a camera placed at the head or foot of the operating table and a probe held by the surgeon. The tip of the probe is displayed on a rendering of an imaging study, which is shown on a monitor adjacent to the patient.

REQUIREMENTS FOR IMAGE-GUIDED NAVIGATION

Spinal navigation requires preoperative or intraoperative imaging systems. The available options include preoperative CT images with or without MR imaging fusion, cone beam CT, intraoperative two-dimensional fluoroscopy, intraoperative three-dimensional fluoroscopy (three-dimensional C-arms rotating around an isocenter),[19] and lately intraoperative CT imaging (O-arm, Medtronic Sofamor Danek, Inc., Memphis, TN; BodyTom, Neurologica Corporation, Danvers, MA; and Airo Mobile, DePuy Synthes, Raynham, MA). Intraoperative MR imaging is used in cranial surgery; however, its use during spine surgery has not been established.[25]

Digital imaging and communications in medicine (DICOM) image sets from CT or MR scans that were obtained before or during surgery are transferred to a computer that displays them. Registration methods that pair imaging with a guidance system have evolved from paired-point systems to surface-recognition software that can automatically register intraoperative fluoroscopy/CT scanners. However, the use of fiducials is not practical in the spine.[20] After the software registers the patient, it is extremely important to establish navigation accuracy (e.g., comparing anatomic landmarks with image data), which normally ranges from 0.42 to 1.08 mm. Errors ± 1 mm are generally accepted.[24]

Red Flag: The use of image guidance requires some planning with respect to the tracker, camera, and monitor placement.

CLINICAL USE

Navigation significantly improves the accuracy of screw placement in all spinal locations.[26-29]

Lumbar Instrumentation

The first successful navigated implantation of pedicle screws was reported in 1995.[19,30,31] In 2007 Kosmopoulos and Schizas[32] analyzed 37,337 navigated and nonnavigated pedicle screws described in 130 articles, including clinical and cadaveric studies. They found that placement of nonnavigated pedicle screws had a mean accuracy of 90.3% compared with a mean accuracy of 95.1% for navigated pedicle screws. In 2014 Sembrano et al[29] showed a 20% change in surgeons' decisions regarding spine procedures that were influenced by intraoperative three-dimensional imaging information; these changes significantly reduced complication rates, optimized surgical results, and prevented reoperations.

Cervical Instrumentation

The use of cervical navigation, especially at the craniocervical and cervicothoracic junctions, is quite helpful in spine surgery.[19,33-37]

Thoracic Instrumentation

The thoracic spine has complex anatomy and small pedicles. Image guidance can be very helpful in this region.[38] Thoracic spine surgery is associated with a significant risk of injury (major complication rate of 15% to 30% in herniated-disc surgeries).[39-41] Navigation has been an important factor in improving these complication rates by giving surgeons real-time feedback during these challenging procedures.

In 2007 Rajasekaran et al[42] treated 33 patients with thoracic deformities and randomly assigned them into navigated and nonnavigated screw insertion groups. They found that 23% of the nonnavigated screws and only 2% of the navigated screws showed pedicle breaches. Despite the breaches, none of the patients in either group had vascular or neurologic injuries.

OTHER USES

Other common procedures that benefit from image-guided navigation are the placement of percutaneous transpedicular screws, transsacral approaches, and screw placement in patients with infection, trauma, and other spinal deformities.[25,43] Image-guided navigation is not routinely used for anterior approaches and is still under development.

> **Red Flag:**
> Advantages of navigation
> - Reduced morbidity
> - Increased implant accuracy
> - Reduced exposure of the surgeon and patient to radiation
> - Feedback for implant placement in all surgical settings with intraoperative three-dimensional navigation
>
> Disadvantages of navigation
> - Repeated verification of landmarks required, with the possibility of losing accuracy
> - Additional time associated with setup
> - Longer surgical times during the learning curve

ROBOTIC ASSISTANCE

Although there is limited evidence favoring robot-assisted pedicle screw placement today,[44] this paradigm will most likely be important in the future of spine surgery.

CONCLUSION

Imaging plays a critical role in the assessment of patients with spinal pain or trauma. However, for the tools to be useful, the appropriate imaging modality and views must be obtained. To plan appropriate treatment, one must carefully correlate imaged abnormalities with the patient's injuries or pain complaints. Physicians should read the films in addition to reviewing the radiologist's reports.

Intraoperative imaging, including technologies incorporating guidance, is rapidly developing and their use is increasing. Image guidance for both conventional and minimally invasive procedures is a powerful tool in spine surgery. It facilitates a surgeon's orientation to unexposed spinal structures, improves precision and accuracy of surgery, and reduces operative time, costs, and radiation exposure. Navigation provides more information to the surgeon than conventional fluoroscopy. Research is needed to determine in which patients and for which types of surgeries these are cost-effective.

REFERENCES

1. Simmons ED, Guyer RD, Graham-Smith A, et al. Contemporary concepts reviews: Radiographic assessment for patients with low back pain. Spine J 3 (3 Suppl):3S-5S, 2003.
2. Boos N, Rieder R, Schade V, et al. The diagnostic accuracy of magnetic resonance imaging, work perception, and psychological factors in identifying symptomatic disc herniations. Spine 20:2613-2625, 1995.
3. Vitaz TW, Shields CB, Raque GH. Dynamic weight-bearing cervical magnetic resonance imaging: Technical review and preliminary results. South Med J 97:456-461, 2004.
4. Herzog RJ, Ghanayem AJ, Guyer RD, et al. Contemporary concepts reviews: Magnetic resonance imaging: Use in patients with low back pain or radicular pain. Spine J 3(3 Suppl):6S-10S, 2003.
5. Webster BS, Bauer AZ, Choi Y, et al. Iatrogenic consequences of early magnetic resonance imaging in acute, work-related, disabling low back pain. Spine 38:1939-1946, 2013.
6. April C, Bogduk N. High-intensity zone: A diagnostic sign of painful lumbar disc on magnetic resonance imaging. Br J Radiol 65:361-369, 1992.

7. Schellhas KP, Pollei SR, Gundry CR, et al. Lumbar disc high-intensity zone. Correlation of magnetic resonance imaging and discography. Spine 21:79-86, 1996.

8. Saifuddin A, Braithwaite I, White J, et al. The value of lumbar spine magnetic resonance imaging in the demonstration of anular tears. Spine 23:453-457, 1998.

9. Smith BM, Hurwitz EL, Solsberg D, et al. Interobserver reliability of detecting lumbar intervertebral disc high-intensity zone on magnetic resonance imaging and association of high-intensity zone with pain and anular disruption. Spine 23:2074-2080, 1998.

10. Ricketson R, Simmons JW, Hauser BO. The prolapsed intervertebral disc. The high-intensity zone with discography correlation. Spine 21:2758-2762, 1996.

11. Guyer RD, Ohnmeiss DD; NASS. Contemporary concepts reviews: Lumbar discography. Spine J 3(3 Suppl):11S-27S, 2003.

12. Guyer RD, Collier R, Stith WJ, et al. Discitis after discography. Spine 13:1352-1354, 1988.

13. Manchikanti L, Benyamin RM, Singh V, et al. An update of the systematic appraisal of the accuracy and utility of lumbar discography in chronic low back pain. Pain Physician 16(Suppl 2):SE55-SE95, 2013.

14. Davis JW, Phreaner DL, Hoyt DB, et al. The etiology of missed cervical spine injuries. J Trauma 34:342-346, 1993.

15. France JC, Bono CM, Vaccaro AR. Initial radiographic evaluation of the spine after trauma: When, what, where, and how to image the acutely traumatized spine. J Orthop Trauma 19:640-649, 2005.

16. MacDonald RL, Schwartz ML, Mirich D, et al. Diagnosis of cervical spine injury in motor vehicle crash victims: How many x-rays are enough? J Trauma 30:392-397, 1990.

17. Holmes JF, Akkinepalli R. Computed tomography versus plain radiography to screen for cervical spine injury: A meta-analysis. J Trauma 58:902-905, 2005.

18. Brandt MM, Wahl WL, Yeom K, et al. Computed tomographic scanning reduces cost and time of complete spine evaluation. J Trauma Inj Infect Crit Care 56:1022-1028, 2004.

19. Ringel F, Villard J, Ryang YM, et al. Navigation, robotics, and intraoperative imaging in spinal surgery. Adv Tech Stand Neurosurg 41:3-22, 2014.

20. Kalfas IH. Image-guided spinal navigation: Principles and clinical application. In Winn HR, ed. Youmans Neurological Surgery, ed 6. Philadelphia: Saunders Elsevier, 2011.

21. Spetzger U, Von Schilling A, Winkler G, et al. The past, present and future of minimally invasive spine surgery: A review and speculative outlook. Minim Invasive Ther Allied Technol 22:227-241, 2013.

22. Karahalios DG, Apostolides PJ, Geldmacher TR, et al. Image-guided spinal surgery. Oper Tech Neurosurg 1:104-112, 1998.

23. Sonntag VKH. Introduction. Oper Tech Neurosurg 1:103, 1998.

24. Merloz P, Lavallee S, Tonetti J, et al. Image-guided spinal surgery: Technology, operative technique, and clinical practice. Oper Tech Orthop 10:56-63, 2000.

25. Moses ZB, Mayer RR, Strickland BA, et al. Neuronavigation in minimally invasive spine surgery. Neurosurg Focus 35:E12, 2013.

26. Assaker R, Reyns N, Vinchon M, et al. Transpedicular screw placement: Image-guided versus lateral-view fluoroscopy: In vitro simulation. Spine 26:2160-2164, 2001.

27. Bostelmann R, Benini A. Computer-navigated pedicle screw insertion in the lumbar spine. Oper Orthop Traumatol 17:178-194, 2005.

28. Holly LT, Foley KT. Three-dimensional fluoroscopy-guided percutaneous thoracolumbar pedicle screw placement. Technical note. J Neurosurg 99:324-329, 2003.

29. Sembrano JN, Santos ER, Polly DW Jr. New generation intraoperative three-dimensional imaging (O-arm) in 100 spine surgeries: Does it change the surgical procedure? J Clin Neurosci 21:225-231, 2014.

30. Nolte LP, Visarius H, Arm E, et al. Computer-aided fixation of spinal implants. J Image Guid Surg 1:88-93, 1995.

31. Nolte LP, Zamorano L, Visarius H, et al. Clinical evaluation of a system for precision enhancement in spine surgery. Clin Biomech (Bristol, Avon) 10:293-303, 1995.

32. Kosmopoulos V, Schizas C. Pedicle screw placement accuracy: A meta-analysis. Spine 32:E111-E120, 2007.

33. Maughan PH, Ducruet AF, Elhadi AM, et al. Multimodality management of vertebral artery injury sustained during cervical or craniocervical surgery. Neurosurgery 73(2 Suppl Operative):271-281; discussion 281-282, 2013.

34. Ogihara N, Takahashi J, Hirabayashi H, et al. Long-term results of computer-assisted posterior occipitocervical reconstruction. World Neurosurg 73:722-728, 2010.

35. Richter M, Cakir B, Schmidt R. Cervical pedicle screws: Conventional versus computer-assisted placement of cannulated screws. Spine 30:2280-2287, 2005.

36. Winegar CD, Lawrence JP, Friel BC, et al. A systematic review of occipital cervical fusion: Techniques and outcomes. J Neurosurg Spine 13:5-16, 2010.

37. Wright NM, Lauryssen C. Vertebral artery injury in C1-2 transarticular screw fixation: Results of a survey of the AANS/CNS section on disorders of the spine and peripheral nerves. American Association of Neurological Surgeons/Congress of Neurological Surgeons. J Neurosurg 88:634-640, 1998.

38. Hott JS, Papadopoulos SM, Theodore N, et al. Intraoperative Iso-C C-arm navigation in cervical spinal surgery: Review of the first 52 cases. Spine 29: 2856-2860, 2004.

39. Ayhan S, Nelson C, Gok B, et al. Transthoracic surgical treatment for centrally located thoracic disc herniations presenting with myelopathy: A 5-year institutional experience. J Spinal Disord Tech 23:79-88, 2010.

40. Huang TJ, Hsu RW, Sum CW, et al. Complications in thoracoscopic spinal surgery: A study of 90 consecutive patients. Surg Endosc 13:346-350, 1999.

41. Quint U, Bordon G, Preissl I, et al. Thoracoscopic treatment for single level symptomatic thoracic disc herniation: A prospective followed cohort study in a group of 167 consecutive cases. Eur Spine J 21:637-645, 2012.

42. Rajasekaran S, Vidyadhara S, Ramesh P, et al. Randomized clinical study to compare the accuracy of navigated and non-navigated thoracic pedicle screws in deformity correction surgeries. Spine 32:E56-E64, 2007.

43. Nottmeier EW, Pirris SM. Placement of thoracic transvertebral pedicle screws using 3D image guidance. J Neurosurg Spine 18:479-483, 2013.

44. Marcus HJ, Cundy TP, Nandi D, et al. Robot-assisted and fluoroscopy-guided pedicle screw placement: A systematic review. Eur Spine J 23:291-297, 2014.

3 ▪ Head and Spine Trauma

Camden Whitaker, Rob D. Dickerman, and Ryan M. Stuckey

In the cervical spine 50% of motion occurs between C1 and C2, with all other motion segments contributing approximately 7%. The C5-6 level, as the fulcrum between the cervical and thoracic spine, is the second most injured area. This chapter will outline the conditions that spine surgeons should be alert for in the emergency department to properly perform an evaluation of a patient with a cervical spine injury.

HEAD TRAUMA (see also Concussions, p. 68)
Clinical Evaluation

- Perform Glasgow Coma Scale (GCS) assessment (Table 3-1, p. 42)
  - Developed for clinical evaluation 6 hr after head trauma occurs
  - Patients should be hemodynamically stable and adequately oxygenated

> **Red Flag:** Hypoxia, hypotension, intoxication may falsely lower the results.

- Closed head injury: High-yield predictors
  - GCS <15, comatose state, prolonged loss of consciousness (LOC), antegrade amnesia, anisocoria, basilar skull fracture, abnormal Babinski's sign, focal motor paralysis, cranial nerve deficit, history of substance abuse.

Table 3-1   Glasgow Coma Scale

Eye Opening	Adults	<1 yr	>1 yr
4	Spontaneous	Spontaneous	Spontaneous
3	To speech	To speech	To speech
2	To pain	To pain	To pain
1	None	None	None

Verbal Response	Adults	Infants
5	Oriented	Coos, babbles
4	Confused	Irritable, cries
3	Inappropriate words	Cries to pain
2	Incomprehensible sounds	Moans to pain
1	None	None

Verbal Response	5 yr	2-5 yr	0-23 mo
5	Oriented/conversant	Appropriate words	Cries appropriately
4	Disoriented/conversant	Inappropriate words	Smiles, coos, cries
3	Inappropriate words	Cries/screams	Inappropriate cries
2	Incomprehensible sounds	Grunts	Grunts
1	None	None	None

Motor Response	Adults	Infants
6	Obeys commands	Spontaneous moves
5	Localizes pain	Withdraws to touch
4	Withdraws from pain	Withdraws to pain
3	Flexion posturing	Abnormal flexion
2	Extensor posturing	Abnormal extension
1	None	None

Pediatric interpretation: Minimum score 3 = worst prognosis; maximum score 15 = best prognosis; scores 7+ = good chance of recovery; scores of 3-5 = potentially fatal, especially if accompanied by fixed pupils or absent oculovestibular responses on elevated intracranial pressure.

Workup

- CT scan
  - Age <2 or >60 years.
  - GCS <15.
  - Loss of consciousness >5 minutes (Cantu grading scale).
  - Change in mental status since injury.
  - Progressing headache.

- Ethanol or drug intoxication may mask symptoms; thus requires CT scan.
- Large cephalohematoma.
- Suspected child abuse.
- Posttraumatic seizure.
- Basilar skull fracture.
- Rhinorrhea or otorrhea.
- Serious facial fractures.
- Unreliable history.
- Decreased level of consciousness.*
- Focal neurologic deficits.*
- Depressed skull fracture or penetrating injury.*
- Occipital fractures are much worse than frontal fractures. Facial bones and the extremities generally buffer the degree of actual skull/brain damage.

- EEG
  - The most common cause of seizures is head injury. An EEG should be considered if clinically indicated.

Treatment/Management

- Nonsurgical
  - Observation
    - CT scan demonstrates no intracranial mass or shift; i.e., no surgical lesion.
    - GCS ≥14.
    - Keep head of bed at 45 degrees; assist with decreasing intracranial pressure.
    - Order neurologic checks by nursing staff q 1-2 hr, depending on level of concern.
    - Prescribe acetaminophen for pain; no heavy narcotics.
    - Avoid giving sedating antiemetics.

---

*Indicates high risk for intracranial injury.

‣ Keep patient NPO until alert.
‣ Repeat CT scan if mental status changes or as scheduled after 24 hours.

■ Guidelines for intracranial monitoring and possible surgical patients
  • GCS ≤8 or an abnormal CT scan or ≥2 of the criteria for high risk of intracranial hypertension despite normal CT scan listed below:
    ‣ Age >40 years
    ‣ Systolic blood pressure <90 mm Hg
    ‣ Decerebrate or decorticate posturing
  • Any patient with an intracranial or extracranial (epidural) lesion will require full neurosurgical evaluation.

Prognosis

■ Based on the Glasgow Coma Scale (Box 3-1)

Box 3-1   Glasgow Coma Scale: Responsiveness After Head Trauma

80% of patients score between 13 and 15 (minor trauma)
  • 3% will deteriorate unexpectedly
10% of patients score between 9 and 12 (moderate trauma)
  • 10% will lapse into coma
  • 20% mortality
  • After 3 months
    − 70% are unable to return to work
    − 90% have memory difficulties
    − 50% permanently disabled
10% of patients score 8 or less (severe trauma)
  • Survivors have a 7% chance of having a moderate disability or good outcome
  • 60% have concurrent major organ damage
  • 40% mortality

INCOMPLETE AND COMPLETE SPINAL CORD FRACTURES
Signs and Symptoms

- Incomplete spinal cord lesions
  - Some function below the area of injury.
  - 90% are central cord, Brown-Sequard, or anterior cord syndrome.

> **Red Flag:** The First National Acute Spinal Cord Injury Study found patients who were treated with methylprednisilone (a 30 mg/kg IV bolus followed by an infusion of 5.4 mg/kg/hr for 23 hours) within 8 hours of injury showed significant neurologic improvement at 6 weeks.

  - ▸ The American Association of Neurosurgeons (AANS) guidelines for treatment of closed spinal cord injury lists methylprednisilone as an option—not as a standard of care or a recommendation because of lack of reproducible evidence.
- Central cord syndrome (most common)
  - ▸ Cause: Elderly persons with degenerative arthritis of cervical vertebrae whose necks are forcibly hyperextended. The ligamentum flavum buckles into the cord, resulting in a concussion or contusion of the central portion of the cord. At the level of injury, flaccid, hyporeflexive; below level, lesion spastic and hyperreflexive.
  - ▸ Affects: Central gray matter, central portions of the pyramidal and spinothalamic tracts.
  - ▸ Symptoms: Quadriplegic with sacral sparing; more symptoms in the upper extremities than in the lower extremities. Fifty percent of patients with severe symptoms will have return of bowel and bladder control, will be able to ambulate, and will regain some hand function.
  - ▸ Prognosis: Overall good prognosis; loss of hand intrinsics is the most frequent sequela.

- Brown-Sequard syndrome
  - Cause: Penetrating lesion; e.g., gunshot, knife wound
  - Affects: Sagittal hemisection of cord
  - Symptoms: Ipsilateral motor paralysis and contralateral sensory hypoesthesia distal to level of injury
  - Prognosis: Best prognosis for recovery
- Anterior cord syndrome
  - Cause: Flexion injuries resulting in cord contusion or protrusion of bony fragments or herniated intervertebral discs into spinal canal. Infarction of anterior spinal artery supplying ventral two thirds of spinal cord.
  - Affects: Anterior portion of spinal cord; gray matter and ventral and lateral white matter tracts.
  - Symptoms: Paralysis and hypoalgesia below the level of injury with preservation of posterior column (position, touch, vibration).
  - Prognosis: Worst prognosis for recovery, even with decompression. Sharp/dull pin prick discrimination indicates better prognosis.
- Additional high cervical spinal cord syndromes
  - Dejeune onion skin pattern of anesthesia of the face caused by damage to the spinal tract of the trigeminal nerve located in the high cervical region.
  - Horner's syndrome: Unilateral facial ptosis, miosis, anhydrosis resulting from a disruption of the cervical sympathetic chain, usually at the level of C7-T2.
  - Posteroinferior cerebellar artery syndrome: Injury to cervicomedullary junction and upper cervical segments.
- The law of the spine (Figs. 3-1 and 3-2)
  If injury zone is from C6-7, then the lowest normal level is C4, because the C5 root exits the cord at a normal level but traverses the injury zone and is injured. This is why half of the patients will improve C5 function without surgery and 66% will improve

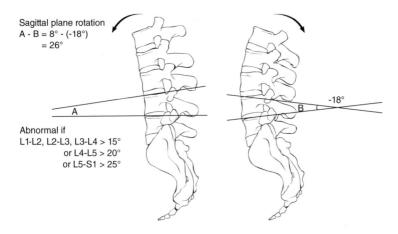

Sagittal plane rotation
A - B = 8° - (-18°)
    = 26°

A

Abnormal if
L1-L2, L2-L3, L3-L4 > 15°
    or L4-L5 > 20°
    or L5-S1 > 25°

-18°

B

Fig. 3-1 Angular instability.

Abnormal if
A > 4.5 mm
or
$\dfrac{A}{B}$ x 100 > 15%

B

A

Fig. 3-2 Measurement to determine vertebral translation or displacement in the lumbar spine. A method for measuring sagittal plane translation or displacement. If the translation or displacement is as much as 4.5 mm or 15% of the sagittal diameter of the adjacent vertebra, it is considered to be abnormal.

with decompression. Also, a patient with an injury at C6-7 will present with flaccid paralysis because the nerve roots are injured as well as the cord. Conversely, a patient with a C8 injury will have spastic paralysis because the nerve root is uninjured but is not receiving information from the injured cord. This stops the negative inhibition of the cord on reflexes and produces spasms.

- Complete spinal cord lesions
  - Total loss of motor and sensation distal to area of injury.
  - Condition persisting greater than 24 hours. Ninety-nine percent of patients will not have a functional recovery.
  - Sacral sparing signs: Persistent perianal sensation, rectal sphincter tone or slight flexor toe movement.
  - Spinal shock.
    - Results from concussive injury to the spinal cord, which causes total neurologic dysfunction distal to the site of injury (flaccid paralysis, absent deep tendon reflex [DTR], hypotension, hypothermia, bradycardia).
    - Usually lasts 24 hours.
    - The end of spinal shock is heralded by the return of the bulbocavernosus reflex. Any reflex can signal the end of spinal shock, but the bulbocavernosus is the most reproducible. No accurate estimates of the patient's prognosis can be made until this reflex has returned.

Clinical Evaluation

- To determine whether the spinal cord injury is incomplete or complete, perform neurologic, sensory, and motor examinations based on the international standards for neurologic and functional classification of spinal cord injury.[1]
  - Neurologic examination
    The neurologic examination has sensory and motor components. Further, the neurologic examination has both required

and optional (though recommended) elements. The required elements are used in determining the sensory/motor/neurologic levels, in generating scores to characterize sensory/motor functioning, and in determining completeness of the injury. The optional measures, though not used in scoring, may add to a specific patient's clinical description.

▸ When the patient is not fully testable

When a key sensory point or key muscle is not testable for any reason, the examiner should record "NT" instead of a numeric score. In such cases, sensory and motor scores for the affected side of the body, as well as total sensory and motor scores, cannot be generated with respect to the injury *at that point in treatment*. Further, when associated injuries such as traumatic brain injury, brachial plexus injury, and limb fracture interfere with completion of the neurologic examination, the neurologic level should still be determined as accurately as possible. However, obtaining the sensory/motor scores and impairment grades should be deferred to later examinations.

▸ Sensory examination: Required elements

The required portion of the sensory examination is completed through the testing of a key point in each of the 28 dermatomes on the right and left sides of the body. At each of these key points, two aspects of sensation are examined: Sensitivity to pinprick and to light touch. Appreciation of pinprick and of light touch at each of the key points is separately scored on a 3-point scale (Fig. 3-3, pp. 50 and 51).

▸ Sensory examination: Optional elements

For purposes of SCI evaluation, the following aspects of sensory function are defined as optional (although they are strongly recommended): Position sense and awareness of deep pressure/deep pain. If these are examined, it is recommended that they be graded using the sensory scale provided herein (absent, impaired, normal). It is also suggested that only one

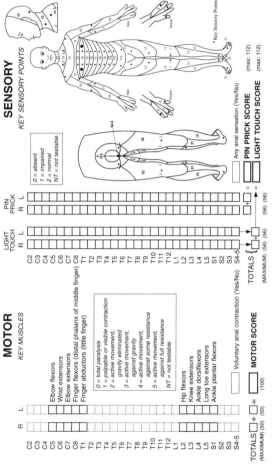

STANDARD NEUROLOGICAL CLASSIFICATION OF SPINAL CORD INJURY

Fig. 3-3 Standard neurologic classification of spinal cord injury: 0 = absent; 1 = impaired (partial or altered appreciation, including hyperaesthesia); 2 = normal; NT = not testable. The following key points are to be tested bilaterally for sensitivity. Asterisks indicate that the point is at the midclavicular line: C2, Occipital protuberance; C3, supraclavicular fossa; C4, top of the acromioclavicular joint; C5, lateral side of the antecubital fossa; C6, thumb; C7, middle finger; C8, little finger; T1, medial (ulnar) side of the antecubital fossa; T2, apex of the axilla; T3, third intercostal space (IS)*; T4, fourth IS (nipple line)*; T5, fifth IS (midway between T4 and T6)*; T6, sixth IS (level of xiphisternum)*; T7, seventh IS (midway between T6 and T8)*; T8, eighth IS (midway between T6 and T10)*; T9, ninth IS (midway between T8 and T10)*; T10, tenth IS (umbilicus)*; T11, eleventh IS (midway between T10 and T12)*; T12, inguinal ligament at midpoint; L1, half the distance between T12 and L2; L2, midanterior thigh; L3, medial femoral condyle; L4, medial malleolus; L5, dorsum of the foot at the third metatarsal phalangeal joint; S1, lateral heel; S2, popliteal fossa in the midline; S3, ischial tuberosity; S4-5, perianal area (taken as one level).

joint be tested for each extremity; the index finger and the great toe of the right and left sides are recommended.

▸ Motor examination: Required elements

The required portion of the motor examination is completed through the testing of a key muscle (one on the right and one on the left side of the body) in the 10 paired myotomes. Each key muscle should be examined in a rostral-caudal sequence. The strength of each muscle is graded on a 6-point scale (Box 3-2).

The muscles detailed in Box 3-3 are to be examined (bilaterally) and graded using the scale defined in Box 3-2. The muscles were chosen because of their consistency for being in-

Box 3-2   Grading Parameters for Muscle Strength

0	Total paralysis
1	Palpable or visible contraction
2	Active movement, full range of motion (ROM) with gravity eliminated
3	Active movement, full ROM against gravity
4	Active movement, full ROM against moderate resistance
5	(Normal) active movement, full ROM against full resistance
NT	Not testable

Box 3-3   Nerve Root Examination

C5	Elbow flexors (biceps, brachialis)
C6	Wrist extensors (extensor carpi radialis longus and brevis)
C7	Elbow extensors (triceps)
C8	Finger flexors (flexor digitorum profundus) to the middle finger
T1	Small finger abductors (abductor digiti minimi)
L2	Hip flexors (iliopsoas)
L3	Knee extensors (quadriceps)
L4	Ankle dorsiflexors
L5	Long toe extensors (extensor hallucis longus)
S1	Ankle plantarflexors (gastrocnemius soleus)

nervated by the segments indicated and their ease of testing in a clinical situation, where testing in any position other than supine may be contraindicated.

For myotomes that are not clinically testable by a manual muscle examination (i.e., C1-4, T2-L1 and S2-5), the motor level is presumed to be the same as the sensory level. In addition to bilateral testing of these muscles, the external anal sphincter should be tested on the basis of contractions around the examiner's finger and graded as being present or absent (i.e., enter "yes" or "no" on the patient's summary sheet). This latter information is used solely for determining the completeness of injury.

▸ Motor examination: Optional elements

For purposes of SCI evaluation, it is recommended that other muscles be evaluated, but their grades are not used in determining the motor score of the motor level. It is particularly suggested that the following muscles be tested: (1) diaphragm (via fluoroscopy), (2) deltoids, (3) abdominals (via Beevor's sign), (4) medial hamstrings, and (5) hip adductors. Their strength is to be described as absent, weak, or normal.

• Sensory and motor scores/levels

▸ Sensory scores and sensory level

Required testing generates four sensory modalities per dermatome: R-pinprick, R-light touch, L-pinprick, L-light touch. These scores are then summed across dermatomes and sides of the body to generate two summary sensory scores: Pinprick and light touch score. The sensory scores provide a means of numerically documenting changes in sensory function. Further, through the required sensory examination the sensory components for determining neurologic level (i.e., the sensory level), zone of partial preservation, and impairment grade are obtained.

▸ Motor scores and motor level

The required motor testing generates two motor grades per paired myotome: Right and left. These scores are then summed across myotomes and sides of the body to generate a single summary motor score. The motor score provides a means of numerically documenting changes in motor function. Further, through the required motor examination, the motor components for determining neurologic level (i.e., the motor level), zone of partial preservation, and impairment grade are obtained.

■ American Spinal Injury Association (ASIA) Impairment Scale

The ASIA grading system was originally developed in 1969 by H.L. Frankel, MD, as a five-grade (A through E) scale for assessing sensory and motor function (Box 3-4). The Frankel scale, as it was called, has been revised several times under ASIA to increase the precise scoring of sensory and motor function.

Box 3-4   ASIA Impairment Scale

A	*Complete* No sensory or motor function is preserved in the sacral segments S4-S5.
B	*Incomplete* Sensory but not motor function is preserved below the neurologic level and includes the sacral segments S4-S5.
C	*Incomplete* Motor function is preserved below the neurologic level and more than half of key muscles below the neurologic level have a muscle grade less than three.
D	*Incomplete* Motor function is preserved below the neurologic level and at least half of key muscles below the neurologic level have a muscle grade greater than or equal to three.
E	*Normal* Sensory and motor functions are normal.

From the American Spinal Injury Association, adapted from the grading system developed in 1969 by H.L. Frankel, MD.

Workup

- Radiography
  - See Tables 3-2 through 3-5 for evaluation of results.[2]
  - To determine cervical pseudosubluxation in children (C2-3), measure the processes anterior border of C1-3. If the C2 border is >1 mm, the injury is not pseudosubluxation.

Table 3-2 C0 to C2 Instability on Radiography

Abnormal	Measure
>8 degrees	Axial rotation C0-1
>7 mm	Additive lateral overhangs C1-2 (check for Jefferson's fracture)
>45 degrees	Axial rotation C1-2
>3 mm	Distance between anterior border of dens and posterior border of the ring of C1, single transverse tear
>5 mm	Bilateral transverse tear
>4 mm	Distance between basion of occiput and top of dens is 4 to 5 mm with flexion-extension views
<13 mm	Distance between posterior margin of dens and anterior cortex of posterior ring of C1 separation Dens tilting of C1 in relations to dens "V" sign

Table 3-3 Cervical Spine Instability on Radiography

Instability	Points
Anterior elements destroyed	2
Posterior elements destroyed	2
Sagittal plane displaced >3.5 mm	2
Sagittal angulation >11 degrees	2
Stretch (+)	2
Spinal cord damage	2
Nerve root impingement	1
Disc narrowing	1
Dangerous loading	1
RESULTS	If >5 points, spine is unstable

Table 3-4 Thoracic/Thoracolumbar Instability on Radiography

Instability	Points
Anterior elements destroyed	2
Posterior elements destroyed	2
Disruptions of costovertebral articulations	1
Radiographically: Sagittal plane displaced >2.5 mm	2
Radiographically: Sagittal plane angulation >5 degrees	2
Spinal cord or cauda equina damage	2
Dangerous loading	1
RESULTS	If >5 points, spine is unstable

Table 3-5 Lumbar Instability on Radiography

Instability	Points
Anterior elements destroyed	2
Posterior elements destroyed	2
Flexion-extension: Sagittal translation >4.5 mm or 15%	2
Flexion-extension: Sagittal plane rotation >15 degrees L1-4; >20 degrees L4-5; >25 degrees L5-S1	2
Resting sagittal displacement >4.5 mm	2
Resting sagittal plane angulation >22 degrees	2
Cauda equina damage	3
Dangerous loading anticipated	1
RESULTS	If >4 points, spine is unstable

- MRI[3]
  - Cord contusion is acutely normal on T1 and bright on T2.
  - Fresh blood becomes bright on both T1 and T2 within several days.
  - Within several weeks, hemosiderin has low T2 signal around the clot.
  - Posttraumatic cysts are low-signal on T1 and bright on T2.

- CT scan
- Aids in fracture classification (Table 3-6)
  - Compression flexion[4] (Fig. 3-4, p. 58)

    Stage 1: Blunting of the anterior-superior margin to a rounded contour. No posterior injury.

    Stage 2: 1+ loss of anterior height with "beak" appearance of the anterior-inferior vertebral body. The concavity of the inferior endplate may be increased.

    Stage 3: 2+ fracture line passing obliquely through the centrum and extending through the inferior subchondral plate. Fracture of the beak.

    Stage 4: Less than 3 mm displacement of the inferior-posterior vertebral margin into the neural canal at the involved motion segment. There is no evidence of additional bone injury between C3 and C4.

    Stage 5: Displacement >3 mm of the posterior portion of the vertebral body fragment posteriorly into the neural canal. The vertebral arch characteristically remains intact. The articular facets are separated, and there is increased distance between the spinous processes. The displacement indicates an injury to both the posterior portion of the anterior ligamentous complex and the entire posterior ligamentous complex.

Table 3-6 Types of Vertebral Fractures

Fracture	Anterior	Middle	Posterior
Compression	X	O	O
Burst*	X	X	X/O
Flexion-distraction†	X/O	X	X
Fracture-dislocation	X	X	X

X = Present; O = not present.

*In a patient with a burst fracture with bilateral laminar fractures and neurologic deficit, there is a 50% to 70% chance of a dural tear.

†A bony flexion-distraction (chance fracture) has better healing potential than a purely ligamentous injury.

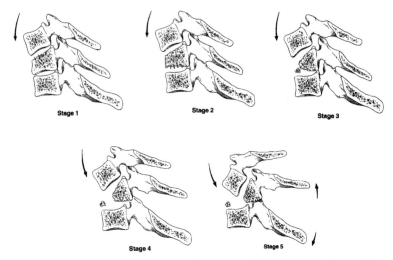

Fig. 3-4   Allen and Ferguson classification of traumatic cervical spine injuries. Compression flexion injury. (From Rizzolo SJ, Cotler JM. Unstable cervical spine injuries. Specific treatment approaches. J Am Acad Orthop Surg 1:57-66, 1993.)

- Vertical compression (Fig. 3-5)

  Stage 1: Fracture of either superior or inferior endplate with cupping deformity. The initial endplate failure is central rather than anterior, no ligamentous injury.

  Stage 2: Fracture of both endplates with cupping deformity. Fractures may exist through centrum but displacement is minimal.

  Stage 3: 2+ centrum is fragmented and its residual pieces are displaced peripherally in multiple directions. The posterior portion of the vertebral body is fractured and may be displaced into the canal. Ligamentous and posterior arch involvement may occur. An intact arch leads to a kyphotic deformity.

Fig. 3-5 Allen and Ferguson classification of traumatic cervical spine injuries. Vertical compression injury. (From Rizzolo SJ, Cotler JM. Unstable cervical spine injuries. Specific treatment approaches. J Am Acad Orthop Surg 1:57-66, 1993.)

- Distractive flexion (Fig. 3-6, p. 60)

  Stage 1: Failure of the posterior ligamentous complex, as evidenced by facet subluxation in flexion and abnormally great divergence of spinous processes at the injury level. Can be accompanied with blunting of the anterior superior vertebral margin to a rounded contour (similar to compression and flexion stage 1 [CFS1]).

  Stage 2: Unilateral facet dislocation. The degree of posterior ligamentous failure may range from partial to complete. Facet subluxation on the opposite side suggests severe ligamentous injury.[1] A small fleck of bone is displaced from the posterior surface of the articular process, which is displaced forward.

  Stage 3: Bilateral facet dislocation with approximately 50% vertebral body with displacement anteriorly. The posterior surfaces of the superior vertebral articular processes lie either snugly against the anterior surfaces of the inferior vertebral articular process or in a perched position.

  Stage 4: Full vertebral body width displacement anteriorly or a grossly unstable motion segment giving the appearance of a floating vertebra.

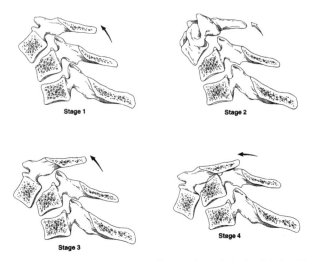

Fig. 3-6 Allen and Ferguson classification of traumatic cervical spine injuries. Distraction flexion injury. (From Rizzolo SJ, Cotler JM. Unstable cervical spine injuries. Specific treatment approaches. J Am Acad Orthop Surg 1:57-66, 1993.)

- Compression extension (Fig. 3-7)
  - Stage 1: Unilateral vertebral arch fracture with or without an-terorotatory vertebral body displacement. An ipsilateral pedicle and laminar fracture resulting in the so-called transverse facet appearance.
  - Stage 2: Bilaminar fractures without evidence of other tissue failure in the cervical motion segments. Typically the laminar fractures occur at contiguous multiple levels.
  - Stage 3: Bilateral vertebral arch corner fractures: articular processes, pedicles, lamina, or some bilateral combination without vertebral body displacement.
  - Stage 4: Bilateral vertebral arch fractures with partial vertebral body width displacement anteriorly.

▸ Stage 5: Bilateral vertebral arch fractures with complete vertebral body width displacement anteriorly. Ligamentous failure occurs at two different levels, posteriorly between the su-
prajacent vertebra and the fractured vertebra, and anteriorly
between the fractured vertebra and the subjacent one.[4] The anterior superior portion of the subjacent vertebral centrum is
characteristically sheared off by the anteriorly displaced centrum.

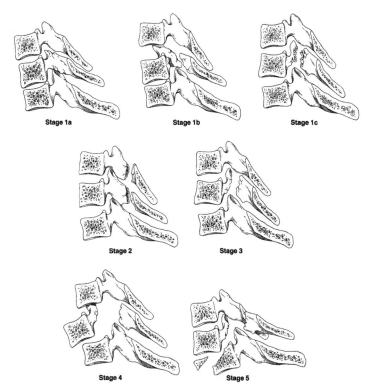

Fig. 3-7 Allen and Ferguson classification of traumatic cervical spine injuries. Compression extension injury. (From Rizzolo SJ, Cotler JM. Unstable cervical spine injuries. Specific treatment approaches. J Am Acad Orthop Surg 1:57-66, 1993.)

- Distractive extension and lateral flexion (Fig. 3-8)
  - ▸ Stage 1: Consists either of failure of the anterior ligamentous complex or a transverse nondeforming fracture of the centrum. When the injury is primarily ligamentous, as it usually is, there may or may not be a brittle fracture of an adjacent anterior vertebral body margin. The radiographic tip-off to the injury is usually abnormal widening of the disc space.
  - ▸ Stage 2: Failure of the posterior ligamentous complex with displacement of the upper vertebral body posteriorly into the spinal canal. Because displacement of the type tends to spontaneously reduce when the head is positioned at neutral posture or in flexion, radiographic evidence of the displacement may be subtle, rarely greater than 3 mm on initial films with the patient supine.

Fig. 3-8 Allen and Ferguson classification of traumatic cervical spine injuries. **A,** Distractive extension injury. **B,** Lateral flexion injury. (From Rizzolo SJ, Cotler JM. Unstable cervical spine injuries. Specific treatment approaches. J Am Acad Orthop Surg 1:57-66, 1993.)

- Lateral flexion
  - ▸ Stage 1: Asymmetrical compression fracture of the centrum plus vertebral arch fracture on the ipsilateral side without displacement of the arch on the AP view. The asymmetrical compression of the vertebral body may appear as an uncovertebral fracture, with some internal collapse of the cephalad vertebral body bone in the region of the uncovertebral joint.
  - ▸ Stage 2: Both lateral asymmetrical compression of the centrum and either ipsilateral vertebral arch fracture with displacement on the AP view or ligamentous failure on the contralateral side with separation of the articular processes.
- Flexion-distraction injury
  - ▸ In the lumbar spine they are associated with 50% incidence of intraabdominal injuries.

Treatment/Management

- Nonsurgical
  - C-collar
  - Halo traction (Box 3-5, p. 64)
  - Acute management of cervical spinal cord injury
    - ▸ Ensure airway: ABCs.
    - ▸ Stabilize neck.
    - ▸ Place Foley catheter.
    - ▸ Maintain perfusion with systolic BP >90.
    - ▸ 100% O_2 saturation via nasal cannula.
    - ▸ Methylprednisolone therapy: Loading dose 30 mg/kg followed by infusion 5.4 mg/kg/hr for 23-48 hours.
    - ▸ Immediate traction reduction for cervical fracture/dislocation.
    - ▸ Surgery if indicated for residual cord compression or fracture instability.
    - ▸ There is no evidence to support the use of methylprednisolone in spinal cord injuries.[5]

Box 3-5 Procedure for Halo Application

1. Determine ring/crown size (hold ring/crown over head and visualize proper fit).
2. Determine vest size (from chest circumference measurement).
3. Pin position:
   a. Anterior pin: lateral two thirds of eyebrows
   b. Posterior pin: 1 cm above ear
4. Shave hair at posterior pin sites and prepare skin with povidone-iodine solution.
5. Anesthetize skin at pin sites with 1% lidocaine hydrochloride.
6. Advance sterile pins to level of skin. Have patient gently, tightly close eyes.
7. Tighten pins at increments of 2 inch-pounds of torque in a diagonal fashion. Seat pins at 8 inch-pounds.
   a. Adults end at 6-8 inch-pounds.
   b. Children <5 yr old end at 4-6 inch-pounds.
   c. Toddlers/infants end at 2 inch-pounds or finger tightness.
8. Apply locknuts to pins. Avoid overtightening.
9. Maintain cervical reduction and raise patient's trunk to 30 degrees.
10. Apply posterior portion of vest and connect to ring/crown with uprights.
11. Recheck fittings, screws, and nuts.
12. Tape tools to vest or keep at bedside (for emergency vest removal).
13. Obtain cervical spine radiographs.
14. Retighten pins once to 8 inch-pounds 48 hours after halo application.
15. Keep pin sites uncovered. Cleanse with hydrogen peroxide every other day or as needed.
16. Looseness of pins may be noted by pain and erythema.
17. Do not retighten after 24 hours; rather, change pin site if necessary.
18. If the neck is immobilized in excessive extension, it can be difficult for the patient to swallow.

From Allen BL Jr, Ferguson RL, Lehmann TR, et al. A mechanistic classification of closed, indirect fractures and dislocations of the lower cervical spine. Spine 7:1-26, 1982.

- Surgical
  - Fusion
    - ▸ New research studies investigating the benefits of stem cells, minocycline, and hypothermia have independently shown positive effects.[6]

ODONTOID FRACTURES
Classification

- Type 1
  - Rare
  - Tip of dens fractured with an avulsion of the alar ligament
- Type 2
  - Most common.
  - Occurs through the base of the odontoid; high nonunion rate.
- Type 3
  - Fracture extends into the body of C2.

Treatment/Management

- Type 1
  - C-collar
- Type 2
  - Surgical options based on fracture angulation, reducibility, vertebral artery, and patient comorbidities.
  - C1-2 cables, C1-2 posterior screws/fusion, anterior odontoid screw, and occipitocervical fusion.
  - New literature has shown that patients undergoing surgery actually do better.[7-9]
  - High complication rate in a halo-vest.[10]
- Type 3
  - Patient will usually heal in a C-collar.

JUMP FACETS AND DISC HERNIATION
Workup

- Radiographs: Besides AP and lateral views, consider oblique and pillar views.
- MRI
  - Indications include patients who are unable to cooperate with serial examinations, intoxication, the need for open reduction, and progression of deficit during an awake reduction.[11,12]

Treatment/Management

- Nonsurgical
  - Application of Gardner Wells tongs
    1. Pins are positioned below the temporalis ridge.
    2. Located 2 cm above the external auditory canal and temporal muscle.
    3. Tongs are secure when pressure pin extrudes 1 mm.

> **Red Flag:** Using tongs, serially increasing traction weight to reduce dislocation has been shown to be safe in patients who are awake and able to cooperate with an examination.[11,12]

  - Reduction attempted by traction administered with the patient under simple sedation. The force applied depends on the level of injury and/or dislocation.[13]
    - The following formula was used to determine the maximum total weight, which was not to be exceeded[13]:

    P = 3 to 4 kg (weight of head) +
                    2 kg per vertebral level away from the cranium

  This weight was obtained by adding increments of 2 or 3 kg followed every half-hour with lateral cervical spine radiographic monitoring. It was suggested to carry out this traction under slight flexion of the neck obtained by placing a cushion under the head. Once the two facets were tip to tip, the neck was reextended. Neurologic status, cardiac rhythm, and BP were monitored at regular intervals. The reduction attempt should not exceed 2 hours of traction.

Red Flag: Herniated discs associated with jump facets in the cervical spine can cause increased neurologic deficit if the patient undergoes surgical open reduction. A few animal studies suggest rapid decompression of the spinal cord may improve neurologic recovery.[11,12]

- Surgical
  - Fusion

Complications

- Vertebral artery injury associated with jump facets
  Vertebral artery stroke can occur with jump facets. The signs of Wallenberg syndrome include (1) ipsilateral loss of pain and temperature sensation in the face, limbs, and trunk, (2) nystagmus, (3) tinnitus, (4) diplopia, (5) contralateral loss of pain and temperature sensation throughout the body, (6) ipsilateral Horner's syndrome, (7) dysphagia, and (8) ataxia.[14] Acute reduction can result in some initial improvement. Vertebral artery injuries can be common in significant cervical facet injuries.[11,14] Stroke may occur immediately after spinal trauma or can be delayed up to a week and sometimes even longer. It also may present concurrent with a spinal cord injury. The occurrence of transient symptoms cranial to the spinal lesion level must be regarded as suggestive of vertebral artery injury, and pending infarction of the vertebrobasilar territory is possible. Doppler ultrasonography and duplex sonography are screening tools for the detection and diagnosis of vertebral artery injuries.[14] Vertebrobasilar infarction after trauma carries a high mortality, and may significantly contribute to the disability of the patient.[11,14]

SPORTS INJURIES OF THE HEAD AND CERVICAL SPINE
Concussions

The diagnosis of a concussion and mild traumatic brain injury has recently received increased attention from scientific researchers, clinicians, and the general public. Both the acute and potential long-term effects of this serious injury have been documented.[15-17] Concussions can occur with any mechanism of trauma to the head, either direct or indirect, and are most commonly sports related. It is estimated that 1.6 to 3.8 million concussions occur annually in sports-related activities.[18] This injury is most commonly associated with American football.

A concussion is defined as a complex pathophysiologic process that affects the brain and is induced by biomechanical forces. This injury results from a direct blow to the head, face, neck, or any other place on the body in which an "impulsive" force is transmitted to the head.

> **Red Flag:** A concussion typically results in a rapid onset of short-lived neurologic impairment that most commonly resolves spontaneously in minutes, but this injury and its associated symptoms can evolve over hours.

- Signs and symptoms
  - May or may not include the loss of consciousness.
  - Somatic (headache), cognitive (the feeling of being "in a fog"), and emotional lability.
  - Amnesia, LOC, unsteadiness, and balance difficulty.
  - Changes in behavior: Irritability.
  - Cognitive impairment: Prolonged reaction times and/or memory changes.
  - Sleep disturbance.
  - The acute signs and symptoms of a concussion are more often related to a functional disturbance rather than to a structural disturbance in the brain. Therefore the findings of neuroimaging studies may appear normal in the acute setting after an injury.

- The resolution of symptoms generally follows a sequential course and is seen within 7 to 10 days in 80% to 90% of patients, but symptoms may be prolonged in certain patients, especially in children and adolescents.[19]
▪ Clinical evaluation
  - The diagnosis of a concussion includes a clinical history, detailed neurologic examination, and a high index of suspicion.
  - The initial history may be best obtained from coaches, spectators, or other athletes who have noted a change in the affected individual.
  - The initial on-field evaluation should include standard first-aid principles, and special care should be given to rule out a potential cervical spine injury. If a cervical spine injury cannot be clinically ruled out on the field, then the individual should be appropriately immobilized until further evaluation is possible.
  - After the initial first-aid care has been given, the athlete can be further evaluated with the Standardized Concussion Assessment Tool (SCAT 3). This has been validated for athletes ages 13 years and older. The Child SCAT 3 is used for those individuals 12 years old and younger.[19]

Red Flag: Because concussions are evolving injuries, the athlete should be monitored for any deterioration during the initial few hours after the injury.

  - After the initial sideline evaluation, the individual must be evaluated in a physician's office or the emergency department. This portion of the evaluation should focus on mental status, cognitive function, gait, and balance. Emergency neuroimaging (CT or MRI) is not warranted unless it is felt that the athlete has sustained a more severe injury that has resulted in a structural abnormality.[19,20]
  - Ultimately, the diagnosis of a concussion is a clinical decision.

> **Red Flag:** Any athlete suspected of sustaining or is diagnosed with a concussion should not be allowed to return to play on the day of injury.[21]

- Neuropsychological (NP) testing
  - ▸ NP testing provides another tool for the evaluation of an individual after a concussion. The role of NP testing is to evaluate the neurocognitive function of the individual.[22] Both pen-and-paper and computer-based evaluations have been shown to effectively evaluate neurocognitive function.[23,24] NP testing is more sensitive than subjective reporting of symptoms. There is generally overlap between clinical symptoms and cognitive recovery, but studies[22,24,25] have shown that cognitive recovery may precede, but more commonly follows, the clinical resolution of symptoms.
  - ▸ There is also evidence that computer-based testing (i.e., ImPACT) provides a more sensitive evaluation than traditional pen-and-paper evaluation. Baseline NP testing can provide a benchmark for the patient, but currently there is no evidence to support the widespread use of baseline NP testing.[19]
  - ▸ NP testing should be used to assist in the clinical evaluation, but should not be the sole basis of releasing an athlete to return to play.

> **Red Flag:** NP testing should be performed within 72 hours after a concussion and then repeated at weekly to biweekly intervals to monitor cognitive recovery.[25]

- Treatment/management
  - Treatment is determined on an individual basis, and standardized testing is available to evaluate whether an athlete can return to the sidelines, class, and/or playing the sport.

- The basis of patient management after a concussion diagnosis is both physical and cognitive rest. A rest period of 24 to 28 hours is recommended after the initial injury.[19] After a short period of rest and resolution of the acute symptoms, the athlete should follow a graduated return-to-play protocol as outlined in Table 3-7.[1] Progression through each level should proceed only if the athlete remains asymptomatic. If the athlete's symptoms return, then the individual should go back to the previous level in the protocol after a period of rest.
- There is new research into the protective roles of progesterone, statin medications, and hypothermia in traumatic brain injury.[26]

Table 3-7 Graduated Return to Game Play

Rehabilitation Stage	Functional Exercise at Each Rehabilitation Stage	Objective of Each Stage
1. No activity	Symptom limited and cognitive rest	Recovery
2. Light aerobic exercise	Walking, swimming, and stationary cycling, keeping the intensity <70% maximum heart rate; no resistance training	Increase heart rate
3. Sport-specific exercise	No head impact activities	Add movement
4. Noncontact training drills	Progression to more complex training drills (e.g., passing drills); may start progressive resistance training	Exercise, coordination, and cognitive load
5. Full-contact practice	After medical clearance, participate in normal training activities	Restore confidence and assess functional skills by the coaching staff
6. Return to play	Return to normal game play	

Data adapted from ASIA website: *http://www.asia-spinalinjury.org*

- Long-term effects
  - Recent attention has been given to the potential long-term effects of a concussion and repeated mild traumatic brain injury. Chronic traumatic encephalopathy (CTE) is the term given to a neurodegenerative disorder that can occur years after an acute head injury.[27,28] Autopsy evaluations of CTE have revealed a specific tauopathy in which neurofibrillary tangles preferentially involve the superficial cortical layers of the brain in the frontal and temporal lobes.[17,29] Clinically, patients with CTE have shown changes in memory, behavior and personality, including depression, irritability, apathy, disinhibition, gait and speech, and parkinsonian-like symptoms. The specific role of a concussion in the development of CTE has not been completely defined, but the relationship varies by sport, duration of exposure, number of injuries, genetic predisposition, and age at initial head trauma.[29]

The Spine and Football Injuries

The cervical musculature, discs, and normal sagittal alignment with lordotic curvature of the cervical spine can withstand significant collision force.[11] Anatomically, the spinal cord in flexion initially unfolds and then elastically deforms with full flexion. Furthermore, during flexion the spinal canal lengthens (the opposite is true for extension: the spinal cord relaxes, folds, and the spinal canal shortens). This lengthening and deformation may explain Lhermitte's sign as the cord is pulled anteriorly over an anterior osteophyte or disc, creating compression of the spinal cord.[11] In football the majority of contact is with a slightly flexed cervical spine. During this slight flexion of approximately 30 degrees, the sagittal alignment or lordosis is flattened and the forces applied to the top of the head are directed at a straight segmented column. The spine is vulnerable in this position and loses its ability to absorb force.[11,30,31] With increasing vertical or axial force to the head and neck in this position, the discs begin to compress and angular deformation and buckling can occur.[11,30,32] This can result in cervical fracture or dislocation. To minimize cervical injuries in football players, the National Football Head and Neck Injury Registry has recommended the following[11,30,31]:

1. No player should intentionally strike an opponent with the crown or top of the helmet.
2. No player should deliberately use the helmet to butt or ram an opponent.

Burners

A "burner" is a unilateral phenomenon, involving injury of the nerve at the root level and brachial plexus. It is commonly seen in football as a "hanging arm." There is a 50% incidence among college football players.[31]

- Workup
  - Radiographs on all players with a complaint
  - EMG on patients with persistent symptoms >2 weeks
- Treatment/management
  - Nonsurgical
    ▸ Observation

> **Red Flag:** The athlete needs to be carefully evaluated for return-to-game readiness.

  - Surgical
    ▸ Fusion: If the condition is a result of dislocation or fracture (see previous discussion)
- Recovery rates[31]
  Grade I: Recovery <2 weeks
  Grade II: Recovery >2 weeks, <1 year
  Grade III: Motor and sensory deficit of >1 year without clinical improvement

- Transient quadraparesis and resumption of sports activities

Red Flag: Return to sports should occur only after symptoms resolve and muscle strength approximates the uninjured side.

If a patient is diagnosed with transient quadraparesis, the timing to return to play remains controversial. There are two prevalent schools of thought. First, Watkins[31] reported no increased spinal cord injury in football players with congenitally narrowed spinal canals. Furthermore, they think it is prudent to give information to the athlete on the risks and complications for football and allow the athlete to make the decision about return to play.[11,31] In contrast, Cantu et al[30] suggested that the loss of cerebrospinal fluid space about the spinal cord may signify an increased risk for future spinal cord injury.[11]

- Signs and symptoms
  - ‣ Injury at cord level.
  - ‣ Always bilateral symptoms: Sensory changes and motor paresis.
  - ‣ Cervical stenosis: Normal is 1.0 and <0.8 is significant stenosis.[33] Stenosis does not increase the risk for development of permanent neurologic injury.
- Treatment/management
  - ‣ Early mobilization and resumption of normal activity immediately after neck sprain have been demonstrated to improve functional outcome and decrease subjective symptoms as measured 6 months after the injury.[11,33]
- Recovery
  - ‣ 10 to 15 minutes, but may take up to 36 to 48 hours.
- Torg et al's recommendations regarding return to play[34]:
  - ‣ Torg ratio = Canal/vertebral body. The smaller the canal, the greater the incidence of recurrence (56%) of transient quadraparesis.

1. Asymptomatic + Torg ratio <0.8 = No contraindications
2. One episode of neuropraxia + Torg ratio <0.8 = Relative contraindication
3. Absolute contraindications
   - MRI evidence of cord injury
   - Degenerative disc at the injured level
   - Ligamentous instability
   - Neurologic symptoms >36 hours
   - Multiple episodes
   - Os odontoideum
   - Healed fracture with canal compromise
   - Any alteration of spinal alignment

KEY POINTS

✦ Hypoxia, hypotension, or intoxication may falsely lower the results of the GCS assessment. The First National Acute Spinal Cord Injury Study found that patients with incomplete spinal cord lesions who were treated with methylprednisolone (a 30 mg/kg IV bolus followed by an infusion of 5.4 mg/kg/hr for 23 hours) within 8 hours of injury showed significant neurologic improvement at 6 weeks.

✦ Using tongs, serially increasing traction weight to reduce dislocation has been shown to be safe in patients who are awake and able to cooperate with an examination.[13,14]

✦ Herniated discs associated with jump facets in the cervical spine can cause increased neurologic deficit if the patient undergoes surgical open reduction. A few animal studies suggest that rapid decompression of the spinal cord may improve neurologic recovery.[13,14]

✦ Athletes need to be carefully evaluated for return-to-game readiness.

✦ Return to sports should occur only after the symptoms resolve and muscle strength approximates the uninjured side.

+ Concussions typically result in a rapid onset of short-lived neurologic impairment that most commonly resolves spontaneously in minutes, but this injury and its associated symptoms can evolve over hours.
+ Because concussions are evolving injuries, the athlete should be monitored for any deterioration during the initial few hours after the injury.
+ NP testing should be performed within 72 hours after a concussion and then repeated at weekly to biweekly intervals to monitor cognitive recovery.[25]

REFERENCES

1. ASIA website: *http://www.asia-spinalinjury.org/home/index.html*.
2. White A, Panjabi M. Spinal Stability: Evaluation and Treatment. AAOS Instructional Course Lectures, vol 30. St Louis: Mosby, 1982.
3. Rothman S. In Capen DA, Haye W, eds. Comprehensive Management of Spine Trauma. St Louis: Mosby, 1998.
4. Allen BL Jr, Ferguson RL, Lehmann TR, et al. A mechanistic classification of closed, indirect fractures and dislocations of the lower cervical spine. Spine 7:1-26, 1982.
5. Hurlbert RJ, Hadley MN, Walters BC, et al. Pharmacological therapy for acute spinal cord injury. Neurosurgery 72(Suppl 2):93-105, 2013.
6. Penha EM, Meira CS, Guimarães ET, et al. Use of autologous mesenchymal stem cells derived from bone marrow for the treatment of naturally injured spinal cord in dogs. Stem Cells Int 2014:437521, 2014.
7. Monaco EA, Weiner GM. Randomized-controlled trial of minocycline for spinal cord injury shows promise. Neurosurgery Feb 72:N17-N19, 2013.
8. Hansebout RR, Hansebout CR. Local cooling for traumatic spinal cord injury: Outcomes for 20 patients and review of the literature. J Neurosurg Spine 20:550-561, 2014.
9. Chapman J, Smith JS, Kopjan B, et al. The AOSpine North America Geriatric Odontoid Fracture Mortality Study: A retrospective review of mortality outcomes for operative versus nonoperative treatment of 322 patients with long-term follow-up. Spine 38:1098-1104, 2013.
10. Harrop JS. Type II odontoid fractures: What to do? World Neurosurg 80:313-314, 2013.

11. American Academy of Orthopaedic Surgeons. Orthopaedic Special Interest Examination 2003. Adult Spine Self Assessment Examination. Rosemont, IL: The Academy, 2003.

12. Botte MJ, Byrne TP, Abrams RA, et al. Halo skeletal fixation: Techniques of application and prevention of complications. J Am Acad Orthop Surg 4:44-53, 1996.

13. Vital JM, Gille O, Senegas J, et al. Reduction technique for uni- and biarticular dislocations of the lower cervical spine. Spine 23:949-954, 1998.

14. Schellinger PD, Schwab S, Krieger D, et al. Masking of vertebral artery dissection by severe trauma to the cervical spine. Spine 26:314-319, 2001.

15. Daneshvar DH, Nowinski CJ, McKee AC, et al. The epidemiology of sport-related concussion. Clin Sports Med 30:1-17, 2011.

16. Bailes JE, Petraglia AL, Omalu BI, et al. Role of subconcussion in repetitive mild traumatic brain injury. J Neurosurg 119:1235-1245, 2013.

17. McKee AC, Cantu RC, Nowinski CJ, et al. Chronic traumatic encephalopathy in athletes: Progressive tauopathy after repetitive head injury. J Neuropathol Exp Neurol 68:709-735, 2009.

18. Langlois JA, Rutland-Brown W, Wald MM. The epidemiology and impact of traumatic brain injury: A brief overview. J Head Trauma Rehabil 21:375-378, 2006.

19. McCrory P, Meeuwisse WH, Aubry M, et al. Consensus statement on concussion in sport: The 4th International Conference on Concussion in Sport, Zurich, November 2012. Br J Sports Med 47:250-258, 2013.

20. Putukian M. The acute symptoms of sport-related concussion: Diagnosis and on-field management. Clin Sports Med 30:49-61, 2011.

21. Lovell M, Collins M, Bradley J. Return to play following sports-related concussion. Clin Sports Med 23:421-441, 2004.

22. Johnson EW, Kegel NE, Collins MW. Neuropsychological assessment of sport-related concussion. Clin Sports Med 30:73-88, 2011.

23. Guskiewicz KM, McCrea M, Marshall SW, et al. Cumulative effects associated with recurrent concussion in collegiate football players. JAMA 290:2549-2555, 2003.

24. Iverson GL, Lovell MR, Collins MW. Interpreting change on ImPACT following sports concussion. Clin Neuropsychol 17:460-467, 2003.

25. Lovell MR, Pardini J, Welling J, et al. Functional brain abnormalities are related to clinical recovery and time to return-to-play in athletes. Neurosurgery 61:352-359, 2007.

26. Harmon KG, Drezner JA, Gammons M, et al. American Medical Society for Sports Medicine position statement: Concussion in sport. Br J Sports Med 47:15-26, 2013.

27. Omalu BI, DeKosky ST, Hamilton RL, et al. Chronic traumatic encephalopathy in a National Football League player: Part II. Neurosurgery 59:1086-1092, 2006.

28. Omalu BI, DeKosky ST, Minster RL, et al. Chronic traumatic encephalopathy in a National Football League player. Neurosurgery 57:128-134, 2005.

29. Gavett B, Stern RA, McKee AC. Chronic traumatic encephalopathy: A potential late effect of sport-related concussive and subconcussive head trauma. Clin Sports Med 30:179-188, 2011.

30. Cantu R, Mueller FO. Catastrophic spine injuries in football (1977-1989). J Spinal Disord 3:227-231, 1990.

31. Watkins RG. Neck injuries in football players. Clin Sports Med 4:215-246, 1986.

32. Thomas BE, McCullen GM, Yuan HA. Cervical spine injuries in football players. J Am Acad Orthop Surg 7:338-347, 1999.

33. Borchgrevink GE, Kaasa A, McDonagh D, et al. Acute treatment of whiplash neck injuries: A randomized trial during the first 14 days after a car accident. Spine 23:25-31, 1998.

34. Torg JS, Vegso JJ, O'Neill MJ, et al. The epidemiologic, pathologic, biomechanical, and cinematographic analysis of football-induced cervical spine trauma. Am J Sports Med 18:50-57, 1990.

4 ▪ Cervical Degenerative Disc Disease

THREE MAIN DIAGNOSTIC CATEGORIES[1]

- Axial neck pain alone
- Cervical radiculopathy (involves compression of a nerve root)
- Cervical myelopathy (involves compression of the spinal cord)

PHYSICAL EXAMINATION: SYMPTOMATIC DEGENERATIVE DISC CONDITIONS

- More pain with neck extension than flexion.
- Pain with flexion is muscle or disc related; pain with extension is facet or foramen related.
- Radiculopathy: Unilateral weakness, nerve root compression, dermatomal sensory changes.
- Spurling's sign: Extension and rotation toward the symptomatic side reproduces the radicular symptoms.

AXIAL NECK PAIN (Figs. 4-1 and 4-2, p. 80)

- Pain that locates in the neck
- No pain in the scapula area or extremities

Signs and Symptoms

- Pain in the neck, headache related

Clinical Evaluation

- Patient has pain with range of motion.
- Patient has more pain with flexion or extension.

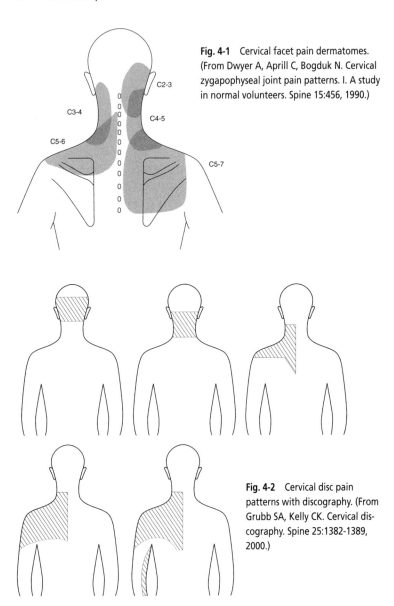

Fig. 4-1 Cervical facet pain dermatomes. (From Dwyer A, Aprill C, Bogduk N. Cervical zygapophyseal joint pain patterns. I. A study in normal volunteers. Spine 15:456, 1990.)

Fig. 4-2 Cervical disc pain patterns with discography. (From Grubb SA, Kelly CK. Cervical discography. Spine 25:1382-1389, 2000.)

Workup

▪ MRI to check for
  • Origin of muscle pain
  • Facet arthropathy
  • Instability
  • Controversial discogenic pain
  • Possible high radicular syndrome from foraminal compression in upper cervical spine

Treatment/Management

▪ Nonsurgical (Box 4-1)
  • Main treatment option
  • Physical therapy
  • NSAIDs
  • Cervical traction
  • Facet injections
  • Controversial: Facet rhizotomies

Box 4-1 Nonsurgical Treatment of Neck Pain, Radiculopathy, and Myelopathy

• Acute painful phase (1-2 weeks): NSAIDs or oral steroids, ice or heat, activity modification, and soft collar or home traction[2]
• Intermediate healing phase (3-4 weeks): Stretching and isometric exercises; consider physical therapy modalities and exercises if the patient is not improving[2]
• Rehabilitation phase (>4 weeks): Cardiovascular conditioning and vigorous strengthening exercise program; 70% to 80% successful outcome expected with 2 to 3 months of conservative treatment[2]
• Collar immobilization to prevent minor injury causing deterioration in neurologic status for patients with myelopathy who are awaiting surgery
• Myelopathy: Reevaluation every 3-6 months to look for deterioration of neurologic function or change in symptoms[3]
• This condition has a lower threshold for surgical intervention than radiculopathy or axial neck pain

- Surgical
  - See Surgical Treatment Options, p. 92.

RADICULOPATHY

Radiculopathy is compression of a cervical nerve root by disc, osteophyte complex, or dynamic instability (Fig. 4-3, pp. 84 and 85).

Signs and Symptoms

- See Fig. 4-3, pp. 84 and 85.
- Pain in scapula and/or extremity.

Clinical Evaluation

- See Fig. 4-3, pp. 84 and 85.
- Check for progressive deficit or disabling deficit.
- Neurologic examination.

Workup

- See Fig. 4-3, pp. 84 and 85.
- If patient exhibits progressive deficit or disabling weakness.
  - Obtain cervical spine series; for inconclusive results, see Fig. 4-3.
  - Flexion-extension radiographs.
  - MRI.

Treatment/Management

- Nonsurgical
  - See Fig. 4-3, pp. 84 and 85.
  - See Box 4-1, p. 81.
  - Collar.
  - Traction.
  - NSAIDs.
  - Heat.
  - Physical therapy for 2-3 weeks.
  - Reevaluation.

- Surgical
  - Indications
    - ▸ Disabling motor deficit at presentation
    - ▸ Progressive neurologic deficit
    - ▸ Persistent radicular symptoms despite at least 6 weeks of conservative treatment
    - ▸ Segmental instability combined with radicular symptoms, significant neurologic deficit, particularly weakness[1,2]
  - Techniques
    - ▸ See Surgical Treatment Options, p. 92.

MYELOPATHY
Signs and Symptoms as an Upper Motor Neuron Disorder

- Global weakness, gait and/or balance problems.
- Hyperreflexia.
- Long tract signs (e.g., Babinski's or Hoffman's reflex and clonus).
- Wasting of shoulder girdle muscles may be evident in patients with stenosis at C4-5 and C5-6.[1]
- Natural history shows slow deterioration over time in typical stepwise fashion and variable periods of stable neurologic function.[1,3]

Clinical Evaluation (Fig. 4-4, p. 86)

- Hoffman's reflex: Hoffman's sign can be elicited by suddenly extending the distal interphalangeal joint of the middle finger. A reflexive finger flexion represents a positive finding.[1]
- Grip-and-release test: The patient is asked to form a fist and to release all digits into extension, rapidly repeating this sequence. A normal response = 20 times/10 sec.[1]
- Paradoxical brachioradialis reflex or inverted radial reflex: Tapping the distal brachioradialis tendon elicits a diminished reflex with a reciprocal spastic contraction of finger flexors if there is cord compression at C6.[1]

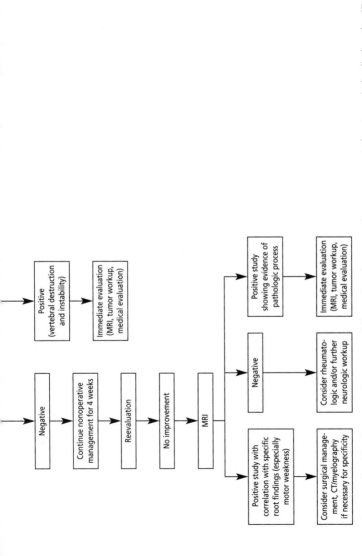

Fig. 4-3 Algorithm for temporal sequences of diagnosis and nonoperative management of acute cervical radiculopathy. *CT,* Computed tomography; *EMG,* electromyography; *MRI,* magnetic resonance imaging; *NSAIDs,* nonsteroidal antiinflammatory drugs. (From Levine MJ, Albert TJ, Smith MD. Cervical radiculopathy: Diagnosis and nonoperative management. J Am Acad Orthop Surg 4:305-315, 1996.)

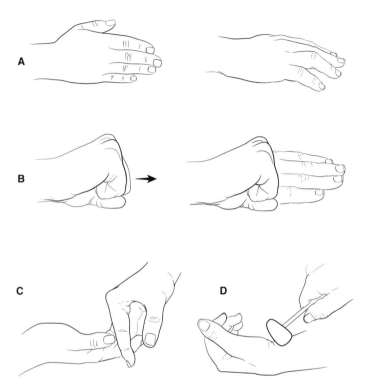

Fig. 4-4 Pathologic reflexes in cervical spondylotic myelopathy. **A,** Finger-escape sign. The patient holds his fingers extended and adducted. In patients with cervical myelopathy, the two ulnar digits will flex and abduct, usually in less than 1 minute. **B,** Grip-and-release test. Normally, one can make a fist and rapidly release it 20 times in 10 seconds. Patients with myelopathy may be unable to do this that quickly. **C,** Hoffmann reflex. Snapping the distal phalanx of the patient's middle finger downward will result in spontaneous flexion of the other fingers in a positive test. **D,** Inverted radial reflex. Tapping the distal brachioradialis tendon produces hyperactive finger flexion. (Modified from Emery SE. Cervical spondylotic myelopathy: Diagnosis and treatment. J Am Acad Orthop Surg 9:376-388, 2001.)

- Scapulohumeral reflex (positive in 95% of patients with a high cord compression): Tapping the tip of the spine of the scapula elicits a brisk scapular elevation and abduction of the humerus if there is high cord compression.[1]
- The proximal motor groups of the legs are involved more than the distal groups, which is the opposite of the pattern with lumbar stenosis.[3]
- Flexion may produce a Lhermitte's sign, an electric-type shock running down the spinal column.[1]
- A hyperactive jaw jerk reflex indicates pathology above the foramen magnum, or in some cases, systemic disease.[1]

Workup

- Disability classification (Table 4-1)

Table 4-1 Nurick Classification of Disability in Spondylotic Myelopathy

Grade	Description
0	Signs of involvement of the spinal cord but gait normal
1	Mild impairment of gait; patient able to work and perform ADLs
2	Mild impairment of gait; patient able to work and perform ADLs
3	Gait abnormality that prevents work and normal ADLs
4	Patient able to walk only with assistance
5	Patient dependent on a wheelchair or bedridden

From Nurick S. The pathogenesis of the spinal cord disorder associated with cervical spondylosis. Brain 95:87-100, 1972. (With permission from Oxford University Press.)
ADLs, Activities of daily living.

- Radiographic considerations
  - Lateral flexion-extension views are helpful to identify compensatory subluxations (hypermobility of motion segments one or two levels above the stiff spondylotic levels).
  - Normal cervical lordosis is 21 degrees.[1]
  - Pavlov's ratio.

- ‣ Sagittal canal diameter divided by sagittal diameter of vertebral body.
- ‣ A ratio of 0.8 or less defines a congenitally narrow spinal canal, which puts the patient at higher risk for cord compression (Fig. 4-5).[4]
- Ishihara index: A comprehensive measurement of the complete cervical lordosis based on the segmental lordosis at each level and then compiled for an overall measurement (Fig. 4-6).
- Loss of cervical lordosis or even kyphosis may accentuate myelopathy (see Fig. 4-6).[3]
- Neck extension decreases the diameter of the spinal canal.[3]
- In patients with spondylosis, a spinal canal measurement on a lateral plain radiograph of 12 mm or less often indicates cord compression.[3]
- If the preoperative cross-sectional area of the cord is <30 mm^2, patients have poorer neurologic recovery.[3]
- Necrosis of central gray matter occurs when the ratio of the midsagittal diameter of the deformed cord to its width (the anterior-to-posterior compression ratio) was less than 1:5.[3] The vascular supply of the gray matter is from the transverse arterioles branching out from the anterior spinal artery system.[3] With flattening of the cord in an anterior-to-posterior direction, these transverse arterioles are subject to mechanical distortion, leading to relative ischemia of the gray matter and medial white matter.[3]
- Ossification of the posterior longitudinal ligament (OPLL): a bar of bone running along the posterior aspect of the vertebral bodies that may be continuous or segmental.
- Instability: Flexion and extension views show >3.5 mm and/or translation >11 degrees of angulation.[3]

Red Flag: Severe radiographic findings that warrant earlier operative intervention include smaller cord area, cord atrophy, signal changes indicative of myelomalacia, or the presence of kyphotic deformity.[3]

Fig. 4-5 Measurement of spinal stenosis. Pavlov's ratio: Spinal cord to vertebral body.

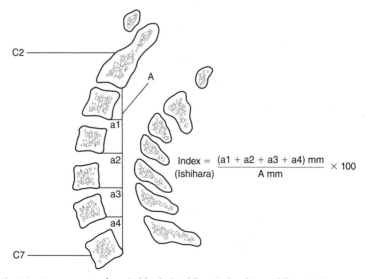

$$\text{Index} = \frac{(a1 + a2 + a3 + a4)\ \text{mm}}{A\ \text{mm}} \times 100$$
(Ishihara)

Fig. 4-6 Measurement of cervical lordosis: Ishihara index. (From Ishihara A. Roentgenographic studies on the normal pattern of the cervical curvature. Nippon Seikeigeka Gakkai Zasshi 42:1033-1044, 1968.)

Treatment/Management

- Nonsurgical
  - See Box 4-1, p. 81.
- Surgical
  - Indications
    - ▸ Progression of signs or symptoms
    - ▸ Presence of myelopathy for 6 months or longer
    - ▸ Canal/vertebral body diameter ratio approaching 0.4
    - ▸ Difficulty walking, loss of balance
    - ▸ Bowel or bladder incontinence
    - ▸ Signal changes within the substance of the spinal cord[1]
  - Techniques
    - ▸ See Surgical Treatment Options, p. 92.

      The goal of surgery in these circumstances is to stop the progression and prevent sudden deterioration after minor injury. The presence of kyphosis dictates an anterior operative approach to adequately decompress the canal and to achieve improvement in the deformity, which augments the direct decompression.[3]

Prognosis

The degree of recovery depends largely on the severity of the myelopathy at the time of intervention.[3]

SPONDYLOTIC MYELOPATHY

This condition is almost always associated with a congenitally narrow spinal canal, which causes symptoms of other compressive pathology. Ossification of the posterior longitudinal ligament can be missed on MRI and is better noted on CT. It is part of the dura and cannot be peeled off of the dura.

Surgical Decision-Making Steps

- Locate compression.

- Check for instability.
- Note alignment: Kyphosis.
- Note level involvement.
- Note adjacent-level disease.

Surgical Treatment/Management (Table 4-2)

- Surgical goal: Decompression without causing instability

Table 4-2   Surgical Treatment of Compressive Pathologies

Compressive Pathology	Surgical Treatment Option
Anterior osteophyte/hard disc	ACDF, ACF
Buckled ligamentum flavum	ACF, LPT
Congenital canal stenosis	LPT
Collapsed disc space	ACDF, ACF
Uncovertebral joint spur	ACDF, ACF
Facet osteophyte	LTM
Disc herniation	ACDF
Special Circumstances	
Spondylolisthesis	ACDF, ACF; can use LPT if fixed
Kyphosis	ACDF, ACF; do not use LPT if >15 degrees of kyphosis
Levels	
1-3 levels	ACDF
3-4 levels	ACF
Multiple levels	LTM/LPT

ACDF, Anterior cervical discectomy and fusion; *ACF,* anterior corpectomy and fusion; *LPT,* laminoplasty; *LTM,* laminectomy.

ADJACENT CERVICAL LEVEL DISEASE

In treating these patients with anterior discectomy and fusion, Hilibrand et al[5] noted 25% of patients had an occurrence of new radiculopathy or myelopathy at an adjacent degenerative level within 10 years of surgery; the highest reoperation rates for the adjacent nonfused segment were for C5-6 or C6-7. Interestingly, patients who had multilevel fusions had a lower incidence of adjacent-segment disease.

Anterior cervical discectomy without fusion has fallen out of favor because of the increased incidence of hypermobility, sagittal plane imbalance, and neck pain on long-term follow-up.[4,5] Controversy still exists about plating, allograft versus autograft, and corpectomy constructs.[4]

> **Red Flag:** The authors concluded that the adjacent degenerative level should be included in the initial fusion in patients with myelopathy or radiculopathy when significant disease was noted.

- See Lumbar Radiculopathy, Chapter 7, for management.

SURGICAL TREATMENT OPTIONS

The following information applies to all three diagnostic categories of cervical degenerative disc disorders.

Monitoring Changes During Spinal Cord Surgery

> **Red Flag:** During the procedure, any change in spinal cord monitoring considered significant should be treated with the same dose of methylprednisolone used for traumatic spinal cord injury (a 30 mg/kg IV bolus followed by an infusion of 5.4 mg/kg/hr for 23 hours).[3]

Anterior Cervical Discectomy and Fusion

- Indications
  - Disc herniation
  - Disc level myelopathy
  - Axial pain with positive discogram[1]
- Compressive pathologies such as disc herniations, spondylosis, and ossification of posterior longitudinal ligaments are anterior to the cord, so direct observation of the pathology and direct removal of the anterior cord compression are possible (Fig. 4-7).[1]

- Compressive pathology limited to one disc space: Anterior discectomy and fusion.
- One or two levels; complications increase significantly with three-level (as opposed to one- or two-level) anterior cervical disc fusion (ACDF).
- "Ideal" tricortical graft[6]
  - Ideal graft thickness is directly related to preoperative baseline disc height.
  - If preoperative disc height is 3.5 to 6.0 mm, the graft should be 2 mm greater than the preoperative disc height.
  - If preoperative disc height is <2.0 mm, the graft should be thicker.
  - If preoperative disc height is >7.4 mm, the graft should be thinner.
- Usual dimensions[6]

Cephalad-caudad	6-10 mm
Medial-lateral	10-15 mm
Anterior-posterior	11-16 mm

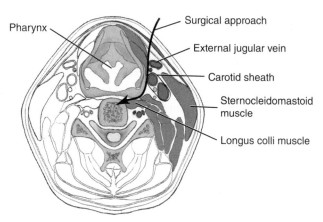

Fig. 4-7 Anterior approach to the cervical spine.

Anterior Cervical Corpectomy: Pathology Behind the Vertebral Body
(see Fig. 4-7, p. 93)

- Cervical myelopathy often has compressive pathology behind the vertebral bodies (e.g., disc, large osteophyte, ossification of posterior longitudinal ligament, cervical kyphosis).[3]
- Use a long anterior plate or buttress plate for two-level corpectomies.
- If three levels or more are to be operated, consider posterior fixation as well (and in osteoporotic patients).
- If three or more levels of stenotic myelopathy are present, consider posterior laminoplasties.
- During corpectomy, the lateral walls of the vertebral body are left intact because they provide protection against vertebral artery injury. The typical midline channel for a corpectomy is 16-18 mm.[3]

Posterior Approach: Posterior Pathologies or Multilevel Stenosis With Neutral or Lordotic Spine

- See Intraoperative Management, Chapter 1, p. 2.
- Patients with preoperative cervical kyphosis are not believed to be candidates for posterior laminectomy or laminoplasty because the cord will stay draped over the kyphotic area, resulting in persistent anterior spinal cord compression (Fig. 4-8).[1] Any posterior decompression procedure is an indirect technique that requires posterior shifting of the cord in the thecal sac to diminish the effect of anterior compression.[3] A kyphotic spine is less likely to allow sufficient posterior translation of the spinal cord to diminish symptoms.[1]
- Laminectomy alone: 20% incidence of later instability with swan neck deformity.
- Laminectomy plus lateral mass fusion: Leaves the neck stiff but allows bilateral foraminotomies.
  - Options for posterior lateral mass screw starting point
    - ▸ Magerl entrance point 1 mm medial and inferior to the center, 25 degrees laterally, and 45 degrees superiorly[6]

▸ An entrance point 1 mm medial to center and 25-30 degrees laterally, and 10-15 degrees superiorly[6]
- Laminoplasty: Offers the advantage of expanding the canal and retaining motion; postoperative neck pain common; patient may still lose 30% motion.
- Several techniques with or without internal fixation.

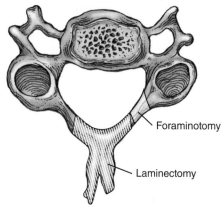

Foraminotomy

Laminectomy

Fig. 4-8 Posterior anatomic location of laminectomy versus foraminotomy in the cervical spine.

Two-Level Cervical Arthroplasty Compared With Two-Level Fusion

- In 2013 Davis et al[7] reported on 225 patients who received the Mobi-C TDR device and 105 patients who received an anterior cervical discectomy and fusion (ACDF).
  - At 24 months only 3% were lost to follow-up.
  - Both groups showed improvements in the Neck Disability Index score and visual analog scale for both the neck and arm. However, the TDR group had significantly greater improvement in the Neck Disability Index score at all time points and significantly greater improvement in neck pain on the visual analog scale.

- The TDR group maintained preoperative segmental range of motion at both treated segments through the 24-month follow-up.
- The reoperation rate was significantly higher for the ACDF group: 11% versus 3%.
- At 24 months the TDR group demonstrated statistically superiority over the ACDF group based on overall study success rates.

Box 4-2   Avoidance and Treatment of Vertebral Artery Injuries

Avoidance
- Mark the midline before dissecting longus colli muscles.
- Frequently reconfirm orientation by referring to midline markings.
- Use the medial uncovertebral joint as a guide for the lateral extent of any dissection or drilling.
- Use caution when dissecting and drilling pathologically softened bones (e.g., tumor, infection).
- Frequently use a measuring standard to confirm orientation (especially when using a microscope).
- If vertebral veins are injured, control bleeding and do not continue dissection further laterally.

Treatment
- Immediately return the patient's head to the neutral position (before attempting to control bleeding).
- Attempt to tamponade bleeding with thrombostatic agents, pressure, and suction. These measures will control most small lacerations effectively.
- If tamponade is unsuccessful, perform direct proximal ligation (may need to unroof anterior bony foramen transversarium immediately beneath the laceration to obtain proximal control).
- Admit the patient to the intensive care unit after surgery for close monitoring of neurologic function.
- Confirmatory radiographic imaging study is mandatory (angiography or magnetic resonance angiography).
- Further management is based on the cause of the abnormality detected (consider reoperation, embolization, heparinization).

Adapted from Heary RF, Albert TJ, Ludwig SC, et al. Surgical anatomy of the vertebral arteries. Spine 21:2074-2080, 1996.

COMPLICATIONS
Vertebral Artery Injuries

See Box 4-2, p. 96.

Pseudarthrosis

Brodsky et al[4,8] reviewed 34 patients who underwent anterior cervical fusion and developed a pseudarthrosis. Seventeen were treated with revision anterior fusion with 75% good results, and 17 were treated with posterior foraminotomy and fusion with 94% good results. Posterior fusion had the most reliable rate of arthrodesis. A neck brace was usually more effective in treating delayed unions identified within the first 3 months after surgery and was unlikely to facilitate pseudarthrosis healing in patients 8 months after surgery.[4,8]

Vocal Cord Paralysis

The cause of vocal cord paralysis during anterior cervical surgery remains controversial. Apfelbaum et al[9] performed 900 anterior cervical surgeries. Thirty patients had vocal cord paralysis, which was permanent in three. These investigators found that retractors placed under the longus colli muscle can compress the laryngeal-tracheal branches within the larynx against the tented endotracheal tube rather than against the recurrent laryngeal nerve, which is extrinsic to the larynx. By deflating/releasing the endotracheal cuff and allowing the tube to recenter itself after placement of the retractors, they were able to decrease the incidence of vocal cord injury from 6.4% to 1.7%. With an incidence of 2%, endotracheal intubation is thought to be the second most common cause of vocal cord injury.[4,9]

Injury of the Superior Laryngeal Nerve: The Professional Singer Dilemma

The superior laryngeal nerve is critical for a professional singer. According to McAfee et al,[10] the nerve can be injured with retraction during vertical extension of common anterior surgical approaches to gain access to the C1-2 and C2-3 levels. They reported on 17 patients in whom a modified submandibular approach was used as an anterior retropharyngeal exposure, with modification of the superior extension of the Smith-Robinson technique, allowing visualization of the superior laryngeal nerve. During this study, no instances of superior laryngeal nerve injury were recorded.

KEY POINTS

✦ When performing a workup for a patient with suspected myelopathy, severe radiographic findings that warrant earlier operative intervention include smaller cord area, cord atrophy, signal changes indicative of myelomalacia, or the presence of kyphotic deformity.[3]

✦ Consider including the adjacent degenerative level in the initial fusion in patients with myelopathy or radiculopathy when significant disease was noted.

✦ During surgical procedures for cervical degenerative disc disorders, any change in spinal cord monitoring considered significant should be treated with the same dose of methylprednisolone used for traumatic spinal cord injury (a 30 mg/kg IV bolus followed by an infusion of 5.4 mg/kg/hr for 23 hours).[3]

REFERENCES

1. Beatty J. Orthopaedic Knowledge Update. Rosemont, IL: American Academy of Orthopaedic Surgeons, 1999.
2. Albert TJ, Murrell SE. Surgical management of cervical radiculopathy. J Am Acad Orthop Surg 7:368-376, 1999.
3. Emery SE. Cervical spondylotic myelopathy: Diagnosis and treatment. J Am Acad Orthop Surg 9:376-388, 2001.
4. American Academy of Orthopaedic Surgery. Adult Spine Self-Assessment Examination. Orthopaedic Special Interest Examination, 2003.
5. Hilibrand AS, Carlson GD, Palumbo MA, et al. Radiculopathy and myelopathy at segments adjacent to the site of a previous anterior cervical arthrodesis. J Bone Joint Surg Am 81:519-528, 1991.

6. An HS, Evanich CJ, Nowicki BH, et al. Ideal thickness of Smith-Robinson graft for anterior cervical fusion. A cadaveric study with computed tomographic correlation [review]. Spine 18:2043-2047, 1993.

7. Davis RJ, Kim KD, Hisey MS, et al. Cervical total disc replacement with the Mobi–C cervical artificial disc compared with anterior discectomy and fusion for treatment of 2-level symptomatic degenerative disc disease: A prospective, randomized, controlled multicenter clinical trial: Clinical article. J Neurosurg Spine 19:532-545, 2013.

8. Brodsky AE, Khalil MA, Sassard WR, et al. Repair of symptomatic pseudoarthrosis of anterior cervical fusion. Posterior versus anterior repair. Spine 17:1137-1143, 1992.

9. Apfelbaum RI, Kriskovich MD, Haller JR. On the incidence, cause, and prevention of recurrent laryngeal nerve paralysis during anterior cervical spine surgery. Spine 25:2906-2912, 2000.

10. McAfee PC, Bohlman HH, Reilly LH Jr, et al. The anterior retropharyngeal approach to the upper part of the cervical spine. J Bone Joint Surg Am 69: 1371-1383, 1987.

5 ▪ Rheumatoid Arthritis of the Cervical Spine

Morbidity and mortality are high after myelopathy develops. All patients with myelopathy will eventually die of the disease.[1] The death rate is high for nonambulatory patients, even those who undergo surgery. Surgery is indicated if the space available for the cord (SAC) is <14 mm.

PREDICTORS OF IMPENDING PROBLEMS[2]

- Subaxial canal at C1-2 <14 mm
- Cranial settling
- Subaxial canal diameter <13 mm

THREE MOST COMMON DIAGNOSES[1]

- Anterior subluxation of C1 on C2 (atlantoaxial instability)
- Cranial settling
- Subaxial subluxation

ANTERIOR SUBLUXATION OF C1 ON C2 (ATLANTOAXIAL INSTABILITY)

This is the most common (49%) and most symptomatic diagnosis; therefore it should be looked for when screening patients. This condition is usually a result of pannus formation at the synovial joints between the dens and the ring of C1 and is also found in 50% of postmortem examinations of patients who have rheumatoid arthritis (RhA).[1]

Workup

- Radiographs
  - Flexion and extension views are used to determine the anterior atlantodens interval (AADI), which is normally <3 mm. A difference of 3.5 mm on flexion and extension views indicates instability; 7 mm implies disruption of alar ligaments; surgery is indicated if the difference is >9 mm.[1,3]
  - Flexion and extension views are used to determine the posterior atlantodens interval (PADI). An interval <14 mm is associated with an increased risk for neurologic injury and requires an MRI.[1,3]
- MRI

Treatment/Management

- Nonsurgical
  - Observation
- Surgical
  - Indications
    - MRI results[1,3]
      - A cervicomedullary angle <135 degrees (normal = 135 to 175 degrees) is an effective measure of cord distortion. This is measured by drawing a line along the anterior aspect of the cervical cord and along the medulla.
      - Cord diameter in flexion is <6 mm.
      - Space available for the cord is <13 mm.
    - Neurologic deficit and intractable pain
      - The PADI has been shown to be a more reliable predictor of whether a patient will develop neurologic compromise.
  - Techniques
    - Laminectomy and fusion
    - Anterior cervical discectomy and fusion
    - Anterior cervical corpectomy

▸ Posterior approach
▸ Laminoplasty

CRANIAL SETTLING

Superior migration of the odontoid (SMO) is the second most common deformity (38%).[1] Dens migration superiorly into the foramen magnum leads to brainstem compression. Ondine's curse: Patients don't wake up from anesthesia.

Workup

- McGregor's line (Fig. 5-1, p. 104) is a line drawn on the lateral view from the hard palate to the base of the occiput. Vertical settling of the occiput has been defined as migration of the odontoid >4.5 mm above McGregor's line.[1,3,4]
- The Ranawat index assesses pathology in the C1-2 segment and is measured on the lateral radiograph by drawing a line from the pedicles of C2 superiorly along the vertical axis of the odontoid until it intersects a line connecting the anterior and posterior arches of C1. A value of <13 mm is diagnostic for vertical settling.[1,3]
- MRI for patients with atlantoaxial subluxation (defined by determining the PADI and the AADI) and any degree of basilar[1,3] invagination.

Treatment/Management

- Nonsurgical
  - Observe patients with isolated, fixed basilar invagination and no symptoms or neural compression.
  - Institute cervical traction for patients with evidence of cord compression.
  - If reduction is possible, use posterior occipitocervical fusion.
  - If reduction is not possible, combine an anterior resection of the odontoid with occipitocervical fusion.

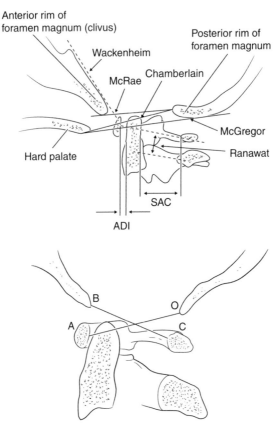

Fig. 5-1 The Powers ratio is determined by drawing a line from the basion *(B)* to the posterior arch of the atlas *(C)* and a second line from the opisthion *(O)* to the anterior arch of the atlas *(A).* The length of the line *BC* is divided by the length of the line *OA,* producing the Powers ratio. (Modified from Lebwohl NH, Eismont FJ. Cervical spine injuries in children. In Weinstein SL, ed. The Pediatric Spine: Principles and Practice, New York: Raven Press, 1994, pp 725-741.)

- Surgical
  - Indications
    - ▸ Subaxial: >3.5 mm of subluxation, or diameter <13 mm[1,3]
    - ▸ See Workup on p. 103.
  - Techniques
    - ▸ Fusion
    - ▸ C1 laminectomy if the brainstem is compressed
    - ▸ Laminectomy and fusion
    - ▸ Anterior cervical discectomy and fusion
    - ▸ Anterior cervical corpectomy
    - ▸ Posterior approach
    - ▸ Laminoplasty
  - Technique considerations
    - ▸ Preoperative traction for 3 to 5 days; halo ring with continued use for 3 months postoperatively or as long as tolerated. If myelopathy resolves while the patient is in traction, fusion can be performed with the patient in that position. If myelopathy does not resolve, reevaluation may be necessary.
    - ▸ In situ fusion
    - ▸ With a long fusion, look for subtle areas of subluxation.
    - ▸ Grob et al[5] noted that pannus resorbs with posterior spinal fusion.

SUBAXIAL SUBLUXATION

Subaxial subluxation may occur after C1-2 fusion and is often an unrecognized, subtle disease. In treating patients it is important to err on the long side of fusion rather than on the short side for patients who do not have rheumatoid arthritis. Subaxial subluxation may also be concurrent and needs to be recognized at the C1-2 fusion.

Workup

- Flexion-extension radiographs
- MRIs

Treatment/Management

- Nonsurgical
  - Bracing or halo traction

Red Flag: This patient population is difficult to treat with these modalities.

- Surgical
  - Indications[1,3]
    - ▸ Mechanical instability
    - ▸ Myelopathy more often than radiculopathy
    - ▸ Posterior atlantodens interval <14 mm in a patient with good function without myelopathy symptoms
    - ▸ Cranial settling
    - ▸ Subaxial canal <12 mm
  - Techniques
    - ▸ Laminectomy and fusion
    - ▸ Anterior cervical discectomy and fusion
    - ▸ Anterior cervical corpectomy
    - ▸ Posterior approach
    - ▸ Laminoplasty
  - Technique considerations
    - ▸ The following instrumentation is recommended:
      - ◆ Bohlman triple wire
      - ◆ Magerl transarticular screws plus posterior fixation
    - ▸ Never go to the other side if you penetrate the vertebral artery.

KEY POINTS

✦ The death rate is high for nonambulatory patients with rheumatoid arthritis of the cervical spine, even for those who undergo surgery.

✦ When treating patients with subaxial subluxation, it is important to err on the longer side of fusion rather than on the shorter side of fusion.

✦ Patients with subaxial subluxation are difficult to treat with nonsurgical modalities, such as bracing or halo traction.

REFERENCES

1. Beatty J. Orthopaedic Knowledge Update 1999. Rosemont, IL: American Academy of Orthopaedic Surgeons, 1999.
2. Boden SD, Dodge LD, Bohlman HH, et al. Rheumatoid arthritis of the cervical spine. A long-term analysis with predictors of paralysis and recovery. J Bone Joint Surg Am 75:1282-1297, 1993.
3. Miller MD. Review of Orthopaedics, 3rd ed. Philadelphia: WB Saunders, 2000.
4. Lebwohl NH, Eismont FJ. Cervical spine injuries in children. In Weinstein SL, ed. The Pediatric Spine: Principles and Practice. New York: Raven Press, 1994, pp 725-741.
5. Grob D, Wursch R, Grauer W, et al. Atlantoaxial fusion and retrodental pannus in rheumatoid arthritis. Spine 22:1580-1583; discussion 1584, 1997.

6 ▪ Spinal Deformities in Pediatric, Adolescent, and Adult Patients

Camden Whitaker and Ryan M. Stuckey

Scoliosis is divided into three categories, each of which requires different treatment interventions: Congenital, idiopathic, and neuromuscular. There are many causes of scoliosis, but adolescent idiopathic scoliosis (AIS) is the most common. AIS is a diagnosis of exclusion, meaning other diseases or causes have to be ruled out first. The condition is hereditary and multifactorial and has no identifiable cause. Causes that have been hypothesized include hormonal (melatonin), brainstem, or proprioception disorders; skeletal muscle abnormalities; abnormal collagen content of discs; fibrilin fibers in ligaments; platelet-calmodulin problems; connective tissue disorders; and growth abnormalities. AIS is defined as a persistent lateral curvature of the spine of more than 10 degrees in the erect position. Although lateral curvature is the main component, it can be associated with rotation of the spine and different plane curvatures. These additional curvatures and rotation make AIS a complex three-dimensional deformity. Treatment is required in 0.2% to 0.3% of patients.

Neuromuscular scoliosis is caused by a wide variety of disorders, including cerebral palsy, Duchenne muscular dystrophy, and myelomeningocele (spina bifida). Each of these categories is very different and requires different treatment interventions than those for AIS.

CONGENITAL SCOLIOSIS

The patient is born with spine curvature caused by a failure of the vertebrae to form or separate from each other.

Signs and Symptoms of Spinal Curvature

- Decreasing order of progression of congenital scoliosis[1]
  1. Unilateral unsegmented bar with contralateral hemivertebra
  2. Unilateral segmental bar
  3. Fully segmented hemivertebra
  4. Semisegmented hemivertebra
  5. Block vertebra

  These are different types of congenital deformities. Depending on the deformity, the progression can be estimated.

Workup

- CT.
- MRI.
- Order additional tests to rule out other anomalies or associated symptoms.

Treatment/Management

- Nonsurgical
  - Bracing: Dependent on age. In most cases bracing is ineffective.
- Surgical
  - Fusion: Anterior or posterior with instrumentation.

INFANTILE IDIOPATHIC SCOLIOSIS
Signs and Symptoms

- Curvature of the spine

Red Flag: Note any intraspinal pathology.

Workup

- Radiographs
- MRI
- Curve measurement (Fig. 6-1)
  - The rib–vertebral angle difference (RVAD) is calculated by subtracting the angle of the rib on the convex side of the curve relative to a line perpendicular to the vertebral body endplate from the angle on the concave side of the curve.[1]
    - ▸ An RVAD of >20 degrees is associated with significant risk of progression, and aggressive treatment is needed to control such curves.[1]

A

SI

Slip angle
(Lumbosacral joint angle)

Slip (%)

B

Convex   Concave

Fig. 6-1   A, Measurements used for evaluation of spondylolisthesis. **B,** The rib–vertebral angle difference (RVAD) is calculated by subtracting the angle of the rib on the convex side of the curve relative to a line perpendicular to the vertebral body endplate from the angle on the concave side of the curve. (**A** modified from Wiltse LL, Winter RB. Terminology and measurement of spondylolisthesis. J Bone Joint Surg Am 65:768-772, 1983. **B** modified from Koop SE. Infantile and juvenile idiopathic scoliosis. Orthop Clin North Am 19:331-337, 1988.)

Treatment/Management

- Nonsurgical
  - Perform casting correction before bracing; if this is ineffective, perform a short segmental anterior spinal fusion across the apex of the curve.[1]
- Surgical
  - A growing rod

ADOLESCENT IDIOPATHIC SCOLIOSIS

AIS is the most common of all scoliosis diagnoses.

- Prevalence (Cobb angle >10 degrees): 25 per 1000 girls-to-boys ratio for curves >25 degrees is 7:1; 3% to 5% have curves >10 degrees (Box 6-1).

Box 6-1 Prevalence: Females/Males

> 11 to 22 degrees: 1.4:1
> >20 degrees: 5.4:1
> >30 degrees: 10:1
> Curve progression in females: 6 to 10 times that in males
> Right thoracic curves are the most common

- Screening: A scoliometer used to measure the angle of trunk rotation (ATR) at the apex of the rib hump provides a useful number on which to base referrals. If the ATR is 5 degrees, only 2% of 20-degree curves are missed, whereas with an ATR of 7 degrees, 12% of 20-degree curves are missed. But most investigators think 7 degrees is an acceptable compromise.[1]
- Natural history: Progression of a curve depends on its magnitude and the skeletal maturity of the patient at the time it is identified. The smaller the curve and the more advanced the skeletal maturity, the less likely it is to increase.

- Risk factors for curve progression: Curve magnitude (>20 degrees), younger age (<12 years), skeletal immaturity (Risser stage 0 or 1) at presentation. Curves <30 degrees at skeletal maturity are not likely to progress. Curves >50 will progress at a rate of 1 degree per year.

PREDICTING WHETHER THE SCOLIOTIC CURVE WILL PROGRESS

The following parameters can predict curve progression and need to be assessed carefully (Fig. 6-2).

- Female sex
- Premenarchal status
- Early Risser sign
- Young age
- Peak growth age: The age after which the rate of growth decreases

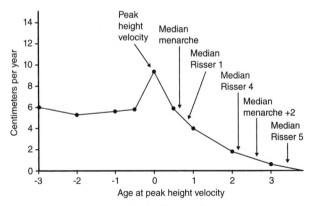

Fig. 6-2 Treatment per curve magnitude. (From Little DG, Song KM, Katz D, et al. Relationship of peak height velocity to other maturity indicators in idiopathic scoliosis in girls. J Bone Joint Surg Am 82:685-693, 2000.)

- Very reliable, not only in terms of progression but also in predicting crankshafting after surgical treatment (Fig. 6-3)
- More reliable than menarchal status
▪ Not predictive: Family history

Clinical Evaluation

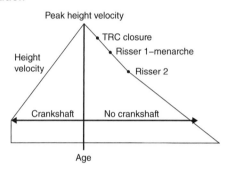

Fig. 6-3 Peak height velocity and its relationship to the crankshaft phenomenon. (From Sanders JO, Little DG, Richards BS. Prediction of the crankshaft phenomenon by peak height velocity. Spine 22:1352-1357, 1997.)

▪ Shoulder evaluation
▪ Waist line asymmetry
▪ Trunk shift
▪ Limb-length inequality
▪ Spinal deformity
▪ Rib rotational deformity (rib hump)
▪ Careful neurologic examination
  - Neurologic examination is especially important with left thoracic curves. An abnormal result warrants an MRI. For example, superficial abdominal reflexes, Beevor's sign (abnormal movement of the umbilicus with a quarter sit-up), indicates rectus abdominis weakness that can result from polio, syrinx, or meningomyelocele.
▪ Determine curve classification

Red Flag: Evaluation should be painless. If it is painful, further testing should be performed to rule out intraspinal pathology.

■ Definition of terms: Structural, major versus minor, location
  • Structural curves
    ▸ Described by their location, structural curves lack normal flexibility; residual 25 degrees and stiff (<30% correction on lateral-bending radiograph). They are termed major (if they have the largest Cobb measurement) or minor. Minor curves can be structural or nonstructural.
  • Thoracic curves
    ▸ The apex of the curve is located between the second thoracic vertebral body and the eleventh and twelfth thoracic intervertebral disc. Proximal thoracic curves have an apex at the third, fourth, or fifth thoracic level. Main thoracic curves have an apex between the sixth thoracic body and the eleventh and twelfth thoracic disc.
  • Thoracolumbar curves
    ▸ Thoracolumbar curves have an apex located between the cephalad border of the eleventh and twelfth thoracic disc and the caudad border of the first lumbar vertebra.
  • Lumbar curves
    ▸ Lumbar curves have an apex between the first and second lumbar disc and the caudad border of the fourth lumbar vertebra.
  • A minor curve is structural if the following criteria are present.
    ▸ A structural proximal thoracic curve has a minimum residual coronal curve on side-bending radiographs of at least 25 (with or without a positive first thoracic tilt) and/or *kyphosis* (from the second to the fifth thoracic level) of at least +20 degrees.
    ▸ A structural main thoracic curve has a minimum residual coronal curve on side-bending radiographs of at least 25 de-

grees and/or *thoracolumbar kyphosis* (from the tenth thoracic to the second lumbar level) of at least +20 degrees.

▶ A structural thoracolumbar/lumbar curve also has a minimum residual coronal curve of at least 25 degrees and/or thoracolumbar kyphosis (from the tenth thoracic to the second lumbar level) of at least +20 degrees, even though sagittal malalignment may be caused by a rotational deformity instead of a true kyphosis.

Adolescent Curve Classifications

- King classification (Fig. 6-4)
  - Type I: Double major.
  - Type II: False double major; lumbar more flexible.
  - Type III: Main thoracic.
  - Type IV: Long C.
  - Type V: Double thoracic.
  - Intended for use only in thoracic curves.
  - Evaluates the coronal plane only.
- Lenke's classification of curve types[2]

First the specific curve type (1 through 6) should be identified (Table 6-1), then the lumbar spine modifier (A, B, or C) and sagit-

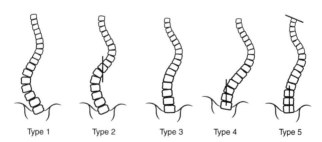

Type 1   Type 2   Type 3   Type 4   Type 5

Fig. 6-4 Adolescent idiopathic scoliosis King curve classification. (From King HA, Moe JH, Bradford DS. The selection of fusion levels in thoracic idiopathic scoliosis. J Bone Joint Surg Am 65:1302-1313, 1983.)

Table 6-1   Lenke Curve Types 1 Through 6

Curve Type	PT	MT	TL/L	Description
1	NS	S*	NS	Main thoracic (MT)
2	S	S*	NS	Double thoracic (DT)
3	NS	S*	S	Double major (DM)
4	S	S*	S*	Triple major (TM)
5	NS	NS	S*	Thoracolumbar/lumbar (TL/L)
6	NS	S	S*	Thoracolumbar/lumbar-MT (TL/L-MT)

From Lenke LG, Betz RR, Harms J. Modern Anterior Scoliosis Surgery. St Louis: Quality Medical Publishing, 2004.
*Major (largest curve).
NS, Nonstructural; *S,* structural.

tal thoracic modifier (−, N, or +) should be defined to determine the exact complete classification of the curve.

- Curve type
  - ▸ Type 1: Main thoracic (MT)
    The main thoracic curve is the major curve, and the proximal thoracic and thoracolumbar/lumbar curves are minor nonstructural curves.
  - ▸ Type 2: Double thoracic (DT)
    The main thoracic curve is the major curve, while the proximal thoracic curve is minor and structural and the thoracolumbar/lumbar curve is minor and nonstructural.
  - ▸ Type 3: Double major (DM)
    The main thoracic and thoracolumbar/lumbar curves are structural, whereas the proximal thoracic curve is nonstructural. The main thoracic curve is the major curve and is greater than, equal to, or no more than 5 degrees less than the Cobb measurement of the thoracolumbar/lumbar curve.

▸ Type 4: Triple major (TM)

   The proximal thoracic, main thoracic, and thoracolumbar/ lumbar curves are all structural; either of the two latter curves may be the major curve.

▸ Type 5: Thoracolumbar/lumbar (TL/L)

   The thoracolumbar/lumbar curve is the major curve and is structural. The proximal thoracic and main thoracic curves are nonstructural.

▸ Type 6: Main thoracic thoracolumbar/lumbar (TL/L-MT)

   The thoracolumbar/lumbar curve is the major curve and measures at least 5 degrees more than the main thoracic curve, which is structural. The proximal thoracic curve is nonstructural.

▸ If the Cobb measurements of the main thoracic and thoracolumbar/lumbar curves are equal, then the thoracic curve is considered the major curve.

• Lumbar spine modifiers (A, B, or C) (Fig. 6-5)

When operative intervention is being considered, the degree of lumbar deformity must be assessed, because it alters spinal balance and affects proximal curves. Three types of lumbar deformity were defined on the basis of the relationship of the center sacral vertical line to the lumbar curve, as noted on the coronal radiograph. The center sacral vertical line should bisect the cephalad aspect of the sacrum and be perpendicular to the true horizontal. Pelvic obliquity secondary to limb-length inequality of <2 cm is ignored, unless the surgeon believes that the pelvic obliquity increases the degree of spinal deformity. In those cases, and when the discrepancy is >2 cm, the coronal radiograph is taken with the appropriately sized lift under the short limb. The center sacral vertical line is extended in a cephalad direction, and the cephaladmost lumbar or thoracic vertebra most closely bisected by the line is considered the stable vertebra. If a

Fig. 6-5   Lumbar spine modifiers. **A,** Type A: Center sacral vertical line (CSVL) between pedicles up to a stable vertebra; zero to minimal scoliosis and rotation of lumbar spine. **B,** Type B: CSVL touches three apical vertebral bodies or pedicles; minimal to moderate lumbar spine rotation. **C,** Type C: CSVL does not touch the apical vertebral body or the bodies immediately above and below the apical disc. (From Lenke LG, Betz RR, Harms J. The Lenke treatment-directed classification system for adolescent idiopathic scoliosis. In Lenke LG, Betz RR, Harms J, eds. Modern Anterior Scoliosis Surgery. St Louis: Quality Medical Publishing, 2004, pp 51-72.)

disc is most closely bisected by the center sacral vertical line, then the vertebra caudad to it is deemed to be the stable vertebra. The apex of a thoracolumbar or lumbar curve is the most horizontal and laterally placed vertebral body or intervertebral disc. Most A and B lumbar modifiers are nonstructural.

▶ Lumbar spine modifier rules

1. Examine the upright coronal radiograph.
2. Accept pelvic obliquity of <2 cm. If >2 cm, you must block out the leg-length inequality to level the pelvis.
3. Draw the center sacral vertical line (CSVL) with a fine-tip pencil or marker. This line will bisect the proximal sacrum and is drawn vertical to parallel the lateral edge of the radiograph.
4. Stable vertebrae are the most proximal lower thoracic or lumbar vertebra most closely bisected by the CSVL. If a disc is most closely bisected, then choose the next caudad vertebra as stable.
5. The apex of the curve is the most horizontal and laterally placed vertebral body or disc.

• Lumbar modifier A (see Fig. 6-5, *A*)
   – CSVL falls between lumbar pedicles up to the level of a stable vertebra.
   – Must have thoracic apex.
   – *If in doubt as to whether the CSVL touches the medial aspect of lumbar apical pedicle, choose type B.*
   – Includes King types III, IV, and V, CSVL between pedicles up to stable vertebra; scoliosis and rotation of lumbar spine: none to minimal.

• Lumbar modifier B (see Fig. 6-5, *B*)
   – CSVL falls between medial border of lumbar concave pedicle and lateral margin of apical vertebral body or bodies (if apex is a disc).
   – Must have a thoracic apex.

- *If in doubt as to whether the CSVL touches lateral margin of apical vertebral body, choose type B.*
- Includes King types II, III, and V.

 ◆ Lumbar modifier C (see Fig. 6-5, *C*)
   - CSVL falls medial to the lateral aspect of the lumbar apical vertebral body or bodies (if apex is a disc).
   - May have a thoracic, thoracolumbar, and/or lumbar apex.
   - *If in doubt as to whether CSVL actually touches lateral aspect of vertebral body (or bodies), choose type B.*
   - Includes King types I, II, and V; double major, triple major, thoracolumbar, and lumbar curves.
   - When curves are assigned lumbar modifier A or B, the lumbar spine should not be included in the arthrodesis unless there is a kyphosis of at least +20 degrees in the thoracolumbar region. The curves that are assigned lumbar modifier C were previously classified as King type I or II, or occasionally as type V, and also include all double major, triple major, and thoracolumbar and lumbar curves. In many cases, when a curve is assigned lumbar modifier C, the lumbar spine probably should be included in the arthrodesis. However, patients who have a 1C or 2C curve may have a selective thoracic arthrodesis, as long as an acceptable balance of the lumbar curve is maintained.

- Sagittal thoracic modifiers (−, N, or +)

 The mean normal sagittal thoracic alignment from the fifth to the twelfth thoracic vertebrae is +30 degrees, with a range of +10 to +40 degrees. Patients who have adolescent idiopathic scoliosis tend to have decreased thoracic kyphosis or even thoracic lordosis in comparison with normal control subjects. The sagittal thoracic modifiers were determined by measurements from the superior endplate of the fifth thoracic vertebra to the inferior endplate of the twelfth thoracic vertebra on a standing lateral radiograph. A minus sign (−) (hypokyphosis) identified a curve of less than +10 degrees, N (normal kyphosis) identified a curve of +10 degrees to +40 degrees, and a plus (+) sign (hyperkyphosis) identified a curve of more than +40 degrees.

Workup

- Radiographs
  - Push-prone
  - Supine
  - AP
  - Lateral
  - Side-bending
  - Standing
  - Lenke's recommendation for his classifications
    - ▸ Workup
      - ◆ Radiographs
        - – Four radiographs of the spine (standing long-cassette coronal and lateral as well as right and left supine side-bending views).
        - – On the basis of this classification, Lenke et al[3] propose that spinal arthrodesis include only the major curve and structural minor curves.
- MRI[4]
  - Note structural abnormalities on radiograph.
  - Excessive kyphosis.
  - Juvenile-onset scoliosis (age >11 years).
  - Left thoracic or thoracolumbar curves.
  - Juvenile-onset scoliosis (age <11 years), infantile onset.
  - Rapid curve progression.
  - Associated syndromes or lower extremity deformities.
  - Neurologic signs/symptoms, including headache.

- Stiff, rigid curves.
- Left thoracic or thoracolumbar curves.
- Cutaneous findings indicative of intraspinal pathology.
- Back pain or other abnormal pain complaints.
▪ CT scan
  - Confirm pedicle width.

Treatment/Management

▪ Nonsurgical
  - Bracing (Table 6-2)
    ▸ Active correction: Three-point fixation with pressure points and relief prevents progression, but does not produce permanent correction.
    ▸ Aim for 50% correction in brace. Prevents curve progression, but does not improve the curve.
    ▸ Success rate is 75% to 80%.
    ▸ The Milwaukee brace: Cervicothoracolumbosacral orthosis (CTLSO) best for T5-12 curves, compared with thoracolumbosacral orthosis (TLSO) for thoracolumbar and lumbar curves.
    ▸ Contraindications to bracing: Growth complete; thoracic lordosis; worsening of thoracic hyperkyphosis in brace; major physiologic reaction; and obesity.

Table 6-2 Treatment for Curve and Growth Rate

Curve (in degrees)	Treatment for Curve and Growth Rate
0-20	Observe for progression
20-25	Brace if progression is documented, and substantial growth remains
25-30	Brace if curve is progressive and growth remains
30-40	Brace if growth remains
40-45	Brace if growth remains (versus surgery)
>50	Surgery

- Surgical
    - ▶ Recommended for all surgical procedures.
  - • Intraoperative spinal cord monitoring (Table 6-3)
    - ▶ Recommended for all surgical procedures.
    - ▶ Stagnara wake-up test: Measures the functional integrity of the complete motor system. Not sensory.
      - ◆ Preoperative phase: The test is discussed with the patient before surgery to ensure that the patient understands what will be required during the surgery.[5]
      - ◆ Intraoperative phase: The anesthesiologist reverses the anesthetic agent and muscle relaxants and wakes the patient to a level of consciousness at which the patient is able to follow commands.[5] The patient is asked to move lower extremity. If a deficit is noted, the patient is reanesthetized and surgery is resumed.
      - ◆ Reliability: Very reliable; having the patient move upper extremity before lower extremity is a good indicator of alertness.[5]

Table 6-3 Electrodiagnostic Findings in Various Peripheral Nerve Disorders

Finding	Root Lesion	Plexus Lesion	Focal Entrapment	Axonal Polyneuropathy	Demyelinating Polyneuropathy
Motor nerve amplitude	± ↓	↓ (focal)	± ↓	↓ (diffuse)	± ↓
Sensory nerve amplitude	Normal	↓ (focal)	± ↓	↓ (diffuse)	± ↓
Distal latency	Normal	Normal	↑ (focal)	Normal	↑ (diffuse)
Conduction velocity	Normal	Normal	↓ (focal)	Normal	↑ (diffuse)
Fibrillations	+ (acute)	+ (acute)	± (severe)	+	±
Large polyphasic MUAPs	+ (chronic)	+ (chronic)	± (severe)	+	±

From Robinson LR. Role of neurophysiological evaluation in diagnosis. J Am Acad Orthop Surg 8:190-199, 2000.
MUAP, Motor unit action potential; +, present; ±, may or may not be present.

- ◆ Validity: 100% accurate in detecting the patient's gross motor movement.[5]
- ◆ Weaknesses: This is a test of gross motor function, not of specific muscle groups. No sensory testing. Moving patient with endotracheal tube (ET) in place to elicit a response; not performed during surgery.
- ▶ Somatosensory evoked potentials (SEPs or SSEPs)[5]
  - ◆ Elicited by stimulating a peripheral mixed (sensory and motor) nerve and recording a response at sites proximal and distal to the level of surgery.
  - ◆ Can be useful in detecting sensory deficits or injury to the spinal cord. During surgery the latency and amplitude of the response are measured and compared with the baseline data (these data are recorded *after* incision to allow anesthetic levels and core temperature to stabilize).
  - ◆ Because of the proximity of the sensory tracts to the motor tracts, if the motor tracts are damaged during surgery, this would also affect the sensory responses, resulting in a diminution or changes in the SSEPs.
  - ◆ The sensory tract used is the tract responsible for proprioception, not sensation of sharp pain, temperature or motor tract function. This means SSEP monitoring only measures potentials produced within the dorsal column of the spinal cord; motor functioning cannot always be assessed via these means.
  - ◆ The vascular anatomy can make evaluation more difficult. The anterior spinal artery perfuses the anterior two thirds of the spinal cord, but the dorsal-medial proprioceptive tract is perfused by radicular arteries. Thus there could be an anterior spinal cord artery injury that is undetected because of the vascular supply of the spinal cord. This false-negative finding indicates that other means of spinal cord monitoring may be necessary to maintain proper sensory and motor functioning.

- Method: During surgery the latency and amplitude of the response are measured and compared with the baseline data.
- Serves as a warning that something might occur, but not an irreversible deficit: Significant when the reduction in amplitude of greater than 50% and/or an increase in latency of 10% relative to baseline values. Amplitude more sensitive.
- Anesthesia: Use IV agents, not inhalational agents.
- Reliability: 1.6% false-positive rate; in the presence of pre-existing neurologic disorders, reliability can be reduced.
- Weakness: If injury involves only the anterolateral columns of the spinal cord, the patient can have a significant postoperative motor deficit in the presence of intact sensory columns.

Red Flag: The use of SEPs with motor evoked potentials is strongly recommended.

- Motor evoked potentials (MEPs)[5]
  - The procedure directly monitors spinal cord motor tract function. This can be done in three ways:
    1. *Electrical stimulation of the motor cortex*
       Electrical method: Subdermal needles are placed in the scalp over the motor cortex; this provides an electrical stimuli that then can be recorded by subdermal needle electrodes placed in the muscles from which data are to be recorded.
       Anesthesia: Isoflurane and neuromuscular relaxants must be discontinued after positioning.
    2. *Magnetic stimulation of the motor cortex*
       Magnetic: The magnetic coil is placed over the motor cortex, which then stimulates the motor cortex, and dis-

tal information can be recorded, as with electrical stimulation.

3. *Electrical stimulation of the spinal cord*
   Spinal cord stimulation by epidural electrodes. Anesthesia does not need to be altered. The responses can be recorded as myogenic or neurogenic.

   - Myogenic response: A muscle contraction that elicits an EMG response. Advantages include large amplitude and reliable latency; disadvantages are that the amplitude and morphology are unreliable. Because of anesthesia, stimulation can cause the patient to move on the table.

   - Based on animal data, a neurologic deficit can affect electrophysiologic data within either 2 minutes for a mechanical injury or 20 minutes for a pure vascular injury.

- EMG testing during surgery[6] (Table 6-4)
  - Higher thresholds indicate intraosseous placement caused by increased resistance to current flow.
  - Rectus abdominis muscles can be used to assess thoracic pedicle screw placement from T6-12.
  - Lumbar pedicle screw threshold values as follows: >8.0 mA confirms intraosseous placement; 4.0-8.0 suggests a potential for pedicle wall defects; and <4.0 is highly predictive of a medial pedicle wall breach. In the cases reported by

Table 6-4 Pedicle Screw EMG Stimulation

Screw Level	Recording Muscle
T6-12	Rectus abdominis
L1-2	Adductors
L3-4	Quadriceps
L5	Tibialis anterior
S1	Gastrocnemius

From Lenke L. Pedicle screw EMG stimulation. Free hand pedicle screw placement [handout]. Seminars in Spine Surgery, 2002.

Tribus,[7] a total of 3.9% of all screws had thresholds of <6.0 mA; however, only 22% of those actually had medial wall perforation confirmed intraoperatively.

- A triggered EMG threshold of 6.0 mA, coupled with threshold values of 60% to 65% decreased from the "average" of all other thresholds in a given patient, should act as a red flag.[6]
- Lenke added that >8 mA confirms intraosseous placement; 4.0-8.0 mA suggests a potential for pedicle wall defects; 4.0 mA is highly predictive of a medial pedicle wall breach.[6]

- Technical considerations for surgery
  - Anatomic variables
    - Pedicle width: CT noted actual pedicle width to be 1 to 2 mm larger than would have been predicted from plain radiographs. Smallest pedicle T5-8 (T6 the smallest).[8] Screw size 4.5 mm in upper thoracic spine, 5.0-5.5 mm in midthoracic spine, 5.5-6.0 mm in lower thoracic spine. Medial wall of thoracic pedicle two to three times thicker than the lateral wall.
    - Neural elements have 1 to 2 mm of space between the medial wall.[8]
    - Dural sac shifted to concavity.
    - Aorta T5-11 is more lateral in a patient with AIS than anterior in a normal spine.[8]
    - Usually SMA syndrome only happens with correction below L1, with large curve correction.
    - There will be more bleeding on the concave side of the spine, because vessels on the convex side are narrowed by the pull of the spine.

- ◆ Anterior spinal fusion approach
    - − Surgeon should selectively go to the convex side, because the concave side is deeper, and larger vessels are present.
    - − Placing the concave rod first will produce a more powerful translation.
- • Indications
    - ▸ Presence of severe deformities (>75 degrees) or to prevent crankshaft (girls <10 years; boys <13 years)
- • Anterior spinal fusion
- • Posterior spinal fusion
    - ▸ Posterior fusion stopping at T10 or 11 can develop segmental kyphosis; this is why the fusion usually should go to T12 or L1.[9]
- • Treatment strategies for specific curve types (Fig. 6-6)[9]
    - ▸ Type 1C curves (N, −): Main thoracic[10]
        - ◆ Posterior instrumentation is placed proximally from the neutrally rotated vertebra above the upper Cobb level and distally to the stable vertebra, which is the vertebra below the Cobb level that is bisected by center sacral vertical line (CSVL).
        - ◆ Anterior instrumentation (same as 1A, 1B) is placed proximally from the upper Cobb level and distally to the lower Cobb level (unless the level below the lower Cobb level had parallel endplates, which would dictate instrumentation).
    - ▸ Type 2 (A, B, C) curves: Double thoracic[10]
        - ◆ Type 2 curves usually require instrumentation and fusion of both curves, which dictates a posterior instrumented fusion.
        - ◆ Selective anterior fusion: Fusing only the main thoracic curve if shoulders are level, no proximal thoracic hyperkyphosis and upper thoracic curve is relatively flexible (<25 degrees).

Level	Cephalad-Caudad Starting Point	Medial-Lateral Starting Point
T1	Midpoint TP	*Junction:* TP-lamina
T2	Midpoint TP	*Junction:* TP-lamina
T3	Midpoint TP	*Junction:* TP-lamina
T4	*Junction:* Proximal third-midpoint TP	*Junction:* TP-lamina
T5	Proximal third TP	*Junction:* TP-lamina
T6	*Junction:* Proximal edge-proximal third TP	*Junction:* TP-lamina-facet
T7	Proximal TP	Midpoint facet
T8	Proximal TP	Midpoint facet
T9	Proximal TP	Midpoint facet
T10	*Junction:* Proximal edge-proximal third TP	*Junction:* TP-lamina-facet
T11	Proximal TP	Just medial to lateral pars
T12	Midpoint TP	At the level of lateral pars

Thoracic Pedicle Screw Starting Points for Anterior and Posterior Fusion

Fig. 6-6   Thoracic pedicle screw starting points for anterior and posterior fusion. *TP,* Thoracic pedicle. (Modified from Lenke L. Thoracic pedicle screw starting points: Free hand pedicle screw placement [handout]. Seminars in Spine Surgery, 2002.)

- ♦ Instrumentation levels: Posterior instrumentation would usually include the upper thoracic curve as well as the main thoracic curve.
- ♦ Distally: Anteriorly, the lower Cobb level, versus posteriorly, the stable level. The use of anterior instrumentation may result in saving proximal as well as distal levels in select cases.
- ▸ Type 3 curves: Double major
  - ♦ Type 3 curves usually require posterior instrumentation and fusion of both curves.

- ◆ A selective anterior or posterior thoracic exception
  - Thoracic selection criteria[9]—correction of the thoracic curve should not exceed the spontaneous correction of the lumbar curve on the push-prone radiograph to avoid decompensation of the lumbar curve.[10]
- ◆ Distal instrumentation levels: Anterior, lower Cobb level; posterior, lower stable vertebrae.[10]
- ◆ Selective thoracic criteria[9]
  - Ratio criteria of MT-to-TL/L 1.2 or greater.
  - Cobb angle.
  - AVT (apical vertebral translation): Curve by the C7 plumb line distance to the midpoint of the apical body or disc.[9] The AVT assessment for the TL/L region is from the midpoint of the apical body or disc to the CSVL. Cages used for sagittal alignment and increased construct stability.[9]
  - Apical vertebral rotation (AVR) is measured at the apex of both curves using Nash-Moe terminology for determining pedicle rotation.[9,11]
  - The vertebral body is divided into six segments and grades from 0 to 4 are assigned, depending on the location of the pedicle within segments (Table 6-5).[11] Because the pedicle on the concave side disappears early in rotation, pedicle on convex side, easily visible through wide range of rotation, is used as standard 5.

Table 6-5   Nash-Moe System for Determining Pedicle Rotation

Grade	Convex Pedicle	Concave Pedicle
Neutral	No asymmetry	No asymmetry
+	Migrates within first segment	May start disappearing
++	Migrates to second segment	May start disappearing
+++	Migrates to middle segment	Not visible
++++	Migrates past midline	Not visible

- Scoliometer measurement[9]
- When the ratio is closer to 2.0 than 1.0, selective thoracic fusion is appropriate. A ratio of ≥1.2 means that one can do an isolated thoracic fusion; AVT is most important.
- Other findings need to be as follows: TL/L flexible; approaching 25 degrees on side-bending radiographs; lack of TL junctional kyphosis (T10-L2 10 degrees).

• Criteria for anterior spinal fusion with implant instrumentation
  - Ability to tolerate single-lung ventilation
  - Short, main thoracic scoliosis segment
  - Small, slender patient
  - Not Scheuermann's kyphosis

• Rod placement
  - To produce kyphosis in the sagittal plane, place the concave rod first.
  - To produce lordosis in the sagittal plane, place the convex rod first.

• Supine radiograph information
  - Position of the spine on the operating table.
  - Pedicles detail better.
  - Best detail of bony elements obtained by supine AP grid film.
  - Large rotational curves should be assessed with supine stagnara radiograph (prominence of the curve hump is flat against the x-ray film).

▶ Type 4 curves: Triple major[10]
  • Instrumentation and fusion of the proximal thoracic, main thoracic, and thoracolumbar/lumbar curves.
  • No selective anterior instrumentation and fusion.
  • These curve patterns would by necessity almost always be treated by posterior instrumentation and fusion.

▸ Type 5 curves: Thoracolumbar/lumbar[10]

  ◆ Isolated anterior or posterior instrumented fusion could be considered.

  ◆ Most commonly treated anteriorly to save a distal level or two in the lumbar spine.

  ◆ Instrumentation from the vertebral level at which one measures the Cobb angle, as long as the lower level has <10 degrees of tilt from horizontal on the reverse side-bending radiograph, and there is <20% rotation in the proposed distal instrumented vertebra.[12]

  ◆ Posterior instrumentation/fusion is a viable option for type 5 curves. Proximal junctional kyphosis has been a complication associated with posterior instrumentation of type 5 curves unless the instrumentation is extended proximally to T9 or T10.5.[10]

  ◆ The distal instrumentation level would normally extend to the stable level. This can result in a fusion that extends one or two levels longer than with anterior instrumentation for the same curve.

▸ Type 6 curves: Thoracolumbar/lumbar and thoracic

  ◆ Generally, both curves will require treatment (posterior approach).

  ◆ Selective anterior or posterior instrumentation and fusion of the thoracolumbar curve can be considered if the ratio of the thoracolumbar/lumbar/thoracic curve is large (1.2) and no thoracic hyperkyphosis, rib prominence, trunk shift, or negative shoulder tilt is present, any of which would necessitate inclusion of the thoracic spine.[10]

  ◆ Obtain a preoperative push-prone radiograph to assess the amount of spontaneous correction of the thoracic curve.[10]

- ◆ The distal anterior instrumented level would be the distal Cobb level, if the lower instrumented level had <20% rotation and was <10 degrees from horizontal on the reverse side-bending radiograph.[12]
- ◆ Posterior instrumentation would need to include the stable level or one level above, usually resulting in a fusion of one or two levels longer than with anterior instrumentation.[10]
- ◆ With either selective anterior or posterior instrumentation, care must be taken to leave a residual thoracolumbar curve to accommodate the thoracic curve and avoid shoulder tilt.[10]
- Satisfactory surgical result
  - ▸ The spine is balanced, the head is centered over the sacrum, and there is no evidence of curve progression at follow-up.
  - ▸ Postoperative pulmonary function.
    - ◆ Owen[5] reported that patients with chest cage disruption noted a decline in pulmonary function at 3 months after surgery, compared with patients without chest cage disruptions, who noted an improvement in pulmonary function at 3 months after surgery.
    - ◆ Regardless of the surgical approach used, postoperative pulmonary function tests returned to preoperative values at 2 years after surgery.[13]

NEUROMUSCULAR SCOLIOSIS
Cerebral Palsy

- ■ Signs and symptoms
  - • Presents with characteristically long sweeping curves.
- ■ Workup
  - • Radiographs
    - ▸ Push-prone
    - ▸ Supine
    - ▸ AP
    - ▸ Lateral

- ‣ Side-bending
- ‣ Standing
- ▪ Treatment/management
  - • See Intraoperative Management, Chapter 1, p. 2.
  - • Surgical[1]
    - ‣ Indications include progressive curves >50 degrees in patient older than 10.
    - ‣ Ambulatory patient should have fusion short of the pelvis.
    - ‣ Both anterior and posterior spinal fusion for crankshafting, severe curve, rigid curve or pelvic obliquity, and loss of sitting balance secondary to curve.

Duchenne and Becker Muscular Dystrophies

- ▪ Signs and symptoms
  - • There is a curve progression of 10 degrees per year once the patient is no longer able to walk.[1]
- ▪ Workup
  - • Radiographs
    - ‣ Push-prone
    - ‣ Supine
    - ‣ AP
    - ‣ Lateral
    - ‣ Side-bending
    - ‣ Standing
- ▪ Treatment
  - • See Intraoperative Management, Chapter 1, p. 2.
  - • Surgical[1]
    - ‣ To allow proper sitting and improve quality of life, posterior fusion with instrumentation should be done as soon as the curve becomes progressive, and before pulmonary function deteriorates beyond a forced vital capacity of <30% to 40%, at which point the patient is no longer a surgical candidate.
    - ‣ Significant pelvic obliquity requires extension to the pelvis.

Myelomeningocele (Spina Bifida)

- Signs and symptoms
  - The incidence of spinal deformity has been correlated with the level of the last intact posterior vertebral arch; the higher the neurologic level, the more likely a spinal deformity.[1]
- Workup
  - Radiographs
    - ‣ Push-prone
    - ‣ Supine
    - ‣ AP
    - ‣ Lateral
    - ‣ Side-bending
    - ‣ Standing
    - ‣ MRI to rule out Chiari malformations, hydrosyringomyelia, and cord tethering[1]
- Treatment/management
  - See Intraoperative Management, Chapter 1, p. 2.
  - Surgical
    - ‣ Anterior and posterior spinal fusion with instrumentation

SCHEUERMANN'S KYPHOSIS
Signs and Symptoms

- Thoracic kyphosis increases throughout life, and in an adolescent is usually between 20 and 40 degrees.[7]
- Patients may present with acute thoracic disc herniations, which because of the deformity may cause neurologic compromise or exacerbation.[14]
- Scheuermann's kyphosis may present with pain just distal to the apex of the deformity located in the paraspinal region.[15]

Clinical Evaluation[7]

- At presentation, when the kyphosis is more than 40 degrees, the patient may need to be evaluated for spinal deformity.

- In the adult population, diagnoses of ankylosis spondylitis, multiple healed compression fractures, tumor, infection, tuberculosis, and postlaminectomy kyphosis need to be excluded.
- In contrast to the adolescent population, spinal deformity in adults can be caused by postural kyphosis, tumor, or infection, in combination with scoliosis, or Scheuermann's kyphosis.
- With severe kyphosis at an early age, the presence of an anterior bar must be ruled out.
- Postural kyphosis can have a sagittal curve as large as 60 degrees, but typical radiographic findings of Scheuermann's kyphosis are not present.
- Because the radiographic findings of Scheuermann's kyphosis are not visible until the onset of puberty, radiographic findings are typically seen in girls earlier than in boys.
- Scheuermann's kyphosis may be separated from familial round-back deformity because Scheuermann's kyphosis has an A-frame deformity with forward bending with a more limited area of involvement while the familial round-back deformity has a more rounded examination.
- Scheuermann's kyphosis might have a histologic origin.
  - ▸ The ratio of collagen to proteoglycan in the matrix of the endplate has been found to be below normal, and this decrease in collagen might result in an alteration in the ossification of the endplate and thus altered vertical growth of the vertebral body.

Workup

- Radiographs
  - Push-prone
  - Supine
  - AP
  - Lateral
  - Side-bending

- Standing
- Postural kyphosis seen on radiographs is correctable on hyperextension exercises, which is not possible with Scheuermann's kyphosis because it is a structural deformity.
- MRI[7]
  - In any presentation of a spinal deformity, if the pain is atypical, an MRI should be obtained to rule out other sources of pain.
  - In any sagittal plane deformity, a severe short segment has the highest risk for neurologic compromise.
  - Schmorl's nodes are herniations of disc material through the vertebral endplate that will lead to a loss of disc height and anterior wedging.
  - Similar to other MRI studies, Paajanen et al[14] reported that 55% of the discs in young adolescents were abnormal on MRI, which was five times that of asymptomatic control subjects.

Treatment/Management

- Nonsurgical
  - Postural kyphosis should be treated with hyperextension exercises.
  - Bracing
    - ▸ Sachs et al[15] suggested 45 degrees as a threshold for initiating treatment for a brace (Milwaukee style). They also demonstrated that of the 120 patients with follow-up of >5 years after discontinuation of the brace, 69% maintained improvement of ≥3 degrees from initial radiographs.
- Surgical
  - See Intraoperative Management, Chapter 1, p. 2.
  - Sachs et al[15] noted that in patients who presented with ≥74 degrees of kyphosis, brace treatment failed in 33% of cases, and these patients needed surgical correction.

- Patients with a kyphosis of ≥75 degrees may be surgical candidates.[15]
- Surgery is indicated for pain, progression, neurologic compromise, cardiopulmonary compromise (usually seen in kyphosis >100 degrees), and cosmesis.[7,14,15]
- Posterior instrumentation and fusion is recommended for patients with a flexible deformity that corrects on hyperextension to less than 50 degrees.[7,14,15]
  - ▸ An anterior release is added to the procedure for patients with more rigid deformities (>75 degrees) and do not correct less than 50 degrees on hyperextension radiographs.[7,14,15]
  - ▸ The anterior release which includes discectomy and interbody fusion is performed on any level that is wedged or has a decreased disc height.[7,14,15]
  - ▸ Posteriorly the instrumentation and fusion should extend from the proximal end vertebra (defined as the most cephalad vertebral body that remains in the concavity of the deformity) to the first distal lordotic disc beyond the transitional zone.[7,14,15]
  - ▸ The surgical correction should not be greater than 50% of the initial deformity or less than 40 degrees.[7,14,15]

Long-Term Prognosis

- The hyperlordosis distal to the thoracic deformity may overload the distal spine causing degenerative disc disease and facet arthropathy resulting in low back pain in adulthood.[7,14,15]

ADULT SCOLIOSIS

Adult degenerative scoliosis develops as a result of asymmetrical narrowing of the disc space and vertebral rotation secondary to the instability caused by disc degeneration.[16-18]

Signs and Symptoms[19]

- Back pain.
- Lumbar curves are usually <40 degrees; rarely progress to >40 degrees.
- Symptoms caused by spinal stenosis either by compression of the nerve roots at the concavity or traction in the convexity of the curve.
  - Collapse in the concavity results in narrowing of the neural foramen between adjacent pedicles. As a result, symptoms on the anterior thigh and leg (resulting from compression of the cephalad and middle lumbar nerve roots) are more common on the side of the concavity of the major lumbar curve.[18]
  - Radiating pain in the posterior portion of the lower extremity is more common on the side of the convexity of the lumbar curve; such pain is due to compression of the caudad lumbar nerve roots and the sacral nerve roots.[18,20]

> **Red Flag:** Unilateral radicular symptoms are much more common on the concavity side.

> **Red Flag:** Most symptoms are consistent with stenosis, with the notable exception that sitting did not relieve leg symptoms.

- As the curve loses its flexibility through the disc degenerative process, the likelihood of curve progression decreases.

> **Red Flag:** Risk factors for curve progression include:
> - Cobb angle >30 degrees
> - Apical rotation greater than grade II (Nash-Moe)
> - Lateral listhesis >6 mm
> - Intercrest line through or below L4-5 disc space

Workup

- MRI or CT/myelogram
- Long standing lateral radiograph for evaluation of sagittal balance
- Supine side-bending films
- Flexion-extension to look for associated instability

Treatment

- Nonsurgical[19]

  80% will respond to conservative treatment.
  - Physical therapy.
  - NSAIDs.
  - Tricyclic antidepressants can help with night pain.
  - Spinal orthoses are used primarily to control symptoms in patients with degenerative scoliosis not to stop progression.
- Surgical
  - See Intraoperative Management, Chapter 1, p. 2.

Indicated for curve progression or stenosis symptoms. 50%-75% improvement of back pain only.

  - Planning
    - ▶ Pelvic parameters
      - ◆ Measurements for the correction of lumbar lordosis and improvement of sagittal balance with regard to the spinopelvic relationship
        - – Normal thoracic kyphosis: −44 degrees ± 19
        - – Normal lumbar lordosis: 53 degrees ± 17
      - ◆ Pelvic tilt
        - – Definition: Vertical line from the femoral head angled with a line from the midpoint of the endplate of S1.
        - – Normal is approximately 20 degrees.
        - – The number 3 is the most important parameter.
        - – How to remember: The vertical line is like the lever at a casino slot machine: "Tilt."

- Demonstrates how the pelvis is compensating for the deformity.
- The more vertical the pelvis (sacrum), the higher the tilt.
- Increase in the pelvic tilt with sacral retroversion and decreases with anteversion: As the pelvis retroverts (the endplate of S1 moves away from the hips), the pelvic tilt increases.
- Changes in lumbar lordosis affect the pelvic tilt.
- Pelvic incidence (PI)
  - Definition: Perpendicular line of the S1 endplate angled with a line from the midpoint of the S1 endplate to the femoral head (or bicoxofemoral = midline between the center of the femoral heads is not lined up on the radiograph).
  - Normal is approximately 55 degrees.
  - This is a morphologic parameter with a fixed value for each individual.
  - The most important parameter is the degree of mismatch between lumbar lordosis and pelvic incidence.
  - Gives the degree of correction needed to restore sagittal balance.
  - Pelvic incidence = lumbar lordosis + 10 degrees (or less).
  - Low pelvic incidence means a vertical sacrum (a more horizontal sacral slope angle or measurement) and loss of lumbar lordosis. It is also associated with a small sacral slope and flattening of the sagittal spine.
  - High pelvic incidence is associated with a large sacral slope and more pronounced sagittal curves.
  - Pelvic incidence = pelvic tilt + sacral slope.
  - Pelvic incidence is the opposite of pelvic tilt: Low pelvic incidence and a high pelvic tilt = loss of lumbar lordosis.
  - The pelvic incidence is used to correct the lumbar lordosis and normalize or improve the pelvic tilt.

◆ Sacral slope
  – Definition: Horizontal line of the posterior S1 endplate point angled with the line of the S1 endplate.
  – Normal is approximately 35 degrees.
  – The smaller the degree, the more vertical the sacrum, demonstrating sacral compensation for the loss of lumbar lordosis or sagittal balance.
◆ The Lafage 3: The three most important pelvic parameters in affecting outcome.[21]
  – Degree of mismatch between lumbar lordosis and pelvic incidence
  – Sagittal vertical axis greater than 5 cm
  – Increase in pelvic tilt
◆ Major concepts in correction
  – The use of compensatory mechanisms to maintain an erect posture, including pelvic retroversion (increasing the pelvic tilt) to retain the vertical position of the trunk when it tilts forward.
  – PI is a fixed parameter, and sagittal alignment requires the use of compensatory mechanisms. Rather than predicting the optimal lordosis, a novel tool is developed to predict a patient's compensatory response to a surgical change of regional alignment (change of lordosis or kyphosis). The significance of this approach is that the predictors are either fixed for a given patient (PI) or controllable by the spine surgeon (lumbar lordosis and thoracolumbar kyphosis), meaning this is a potentially useful tool to predict a patient's postoperative compensation.
  – By surgically correcting lumbar lordosis, the surgeon not only can restore the sagittal curvature, but also correct the pelvic retroversion (pelvic tilt) while restoring global sagittal alignment (sagittal vertical axis).

- Two key parameters in the setting of sagittal balance (pelvic tilt and sagittal vertical axis) can be predicted from a morphologic parameter (PI) and parameters modifiable through surgical correction (lumbar lordosis and thoracolumbar kyphosis).
- By using the pelvic parameters to understand the loss of spinal alignment, the surgeon can determine the correction needed for the thoracic and lumbar spine. This surgical correction restores sagittal balance and reduces the compensatory pelvic mechanisms to normal.
  □ Sagittal vertical axis
    ○ Definition: Distance measured from the C7 plumb line to the posterior point of the S1 endplate.
    ○ Normal is less than 5 cm.
    ○ Second most important parameter in sagittal balance.
    ○ Indicates global sagittal balance.
  □ T1 spinopelvic inclination[22]
    ○ Definition: Vertical line from T1 to the femoral head angled with a vertical line.
    ○ Normal is −4 degrees.
    ○ Most highly correlated with clinical outcome (Lafage).
    ○ A measurement of global spinopelvic alignment.
  □ T9 spinopelvic inclination[22]
    ○ Normal is −14 degrees.
    ○ Definition: A vertical line from T9 to the femoral head angled with a vertical line.
    ○ An indicator of the center of gravity of body parts above the femoral heads.
- ◆ Spondylolisthesis sacral measurements
  - Percentage of slip
    □ Distance between a line parallel to the posterior portion of the S1 vertebral body and a line parallel to the posterior portion of the L5 body = 1

- □ AP distance of L5 = 2
- □ One half = percent slip
  - – Slip angle
    - □ Definition: S1 endplate line angle with the inferior L5 endplate line.
    - □ 40 degrees needs correction.
    - □ Correction of slip is more about correcting the angle rather than the reduction, analogous to correction of a femur fracture in a child.
  - – Compensatory mechanisms and effect of age on sagittal balance in spondylolisthesis
    - □ Younger population (less than 45 years of age): Compensate by hyperlordosis above the spondylolisthesis for loss of sagittal balance.
    - □ Older population: Pelvic retroversion appears to be a secondary compensatory mechanism that is adaptive with patients with a stiffer spine.
    - □ When the extent of pelvic retroversion is reached, hip and knee flexion may occur, representing the third compensatory mechanism.
- Fusion with decompression[23]
  - ▶ Indications for fusion to treat scoliosis: Curve >35 degrees, lateral listhesis, and documented curve progression.[16,17]
  - ▶ Curve progression.
  - ▶ More than 50% curve correction on supine side-bending films has been achieved.
  - ▶ Need to distract pedicles on concavity causing compression of nerve root.
  - ▶ Loss of lumbar lordosis.
  - ▶ Fixed lateral listhesis.
  - ▶ Wide intraoperative decompression.

- Lumbopelvic fixation
  - ▸ Long spinal fusions are often necessary in disorders of the spine, including adult and pediatric deformities, L5-S1 spondylolisthesis, revision laminectomy and decompression, tumor surgery, neuromuscular scoliosis, trauma including spinopelvic dissociation, and in patients with poor bone quality. The complex anatomy and large biomechanical forces at the lumbosacral junction, poor bone quality in the sacrum, and large diameter of the sacral pedicles increase the risks of failure at the distal end of long constructs.[24]
  - ▸ Kim et al[25] reported a 24% pseudarthrosis rate at L5-S1 at the end of the long constructs in adult scoliosis surgery. This can lead to S1 screw pullout or rod breakage and failure of the long construct.
  - ▸ Pseudarthrosis at L5-S1 has resulted in poor clinical outcomes.[26-28] To improve the fusion rate, Tsuchiya et al[27] recommended lumbosacral fixation, including the L5-S1 interbody, S1 pedicle screws, and iliac fixation, in constructs extending proximal to L2.
  - ▸ Different options exist for lumbopelvic fixation, and improved lumbopelvic fixation has been noted with the use of threaded iliac screws compared with the smooth rods used in the original Galveston technique. Threaded iliac screws show increased pullout strength and provide a biomechanical advantage, extending a point of fixation anterior to the lumbosacral pivot point. It has been shown that the addition of iliac screws to long constructs protects the S1 screws from pullout, decreases lumbosacral motion, and decreases the pseudarthrosis rate at L5-S1.[27,29] The use of "complete lumbosacral fixation" has shown primary fusion rates of greater than 95% at L5-S1.[29] Iliac screws are placed through a starting point at the posterior superior iliac spine and advanced between the inner

and outer tables of the ilium directed just superior to the greater sciatic notch. Screw diameters range between 6.5 and 8.5 mm, and the length can extend to greater than 100 mm.

▸ Although iliac screws show improved fusion rates and clinical outcomes when added to long constructs, there are potential downsides to the use of the threaded iliac screw. Implant prominence, added muscle dissection, disruption of the skin and muscle vascularity leading to wound breakdown, the need for placement of offset rod connectors, decreased volume of potential autogenous bone graft, disruption of the sacroiliac joint, and the need for implant removal have been described.[25,30,31]

▸ Kim et al[25] described the addition of bicortical, bitriangulated S2 screws to the distal end of the long construct to protect the S1 screws and improve lumbosacral fixation. The starting point of this screw is located at the midpoint of the line bisecting the S1 and S2 dorsal foramen and the bridge of bone that extends between the S1 and S2 foramen. The screw is then directed perpendicular to the dorsal cortex of the sacrum angled lateral 30 to 35 degrees and cephalad 15 to 20 degrees. This trajectory advances the screw parallel to the sacroiliac joint. The screw is advanced into the anterior cortical bone. In the biomechanical study the authors found that the S1/bicortical, bitriangulated S2 construct was biomechanically equivalent to the S1–iliac screw construct, but the S1–iliac screw construct showed a greater resistance to screw loosening.

▸ Another alternative to traditional iliac screws for lumbopelvic fixation is the S2 alar iliac screw. This technique has been described as both open and percutaneous.[31-33] The starting point for this screw is 25 mm inferior to the superior endplate of S1 and 22 mm lateral to the midline at S2.[31] This has also been described as 1 mm inferior and lateral to the dorsal foramen of

S1.[32] The trajectory is 40 degrees lateral in the transverse plane and 40 degrees caudal in the sagittal plane directed toward the greater trochanter. Radiographically, the trajectory of the screw projects just superior to the greater sciatic notch on the AP radiograph of the pelvis. The starting point is 15 mm deeper from the skin than that of the traditional iliac screw. The potential screw length is up to 100 mm, but studies have shown that a 65 mm S2 alar iliac screw is biomechanically similar to 80 and 90 mm S2 alar iliac screws with offset connectors.[32] The S2 alar iliac screw addresses some of the potential problems associated with traditional iliac screws noted previously. The instrumentation is in line with the proximal aspect of the construct and S1 screws, limiting further muscle dissection and skin incisions. The starting point sits deeper than the posterior superior iliac spine, decreasing implant prominence, and it does not interfere with iliac crest harvest. Similar to the traditional iliac screw, the S2 alar iliac screw crosses the sacroiliac, but the clinical significance has not yet been well defined.

KEY POINTS

+ When diagnosing infantile idiopathic scoliosis, one should note any intraspinal pathology.

+ When the surgeon is assessing the patient to predict whether the scoliotic curve will progress, the evaluation should be painless. If it is painful, further testing should be performed to rule out intraspinal pathology.

+ The use of somatosensory evoked potentials with motor evoked potentials is strongly recommended.

+ When an EMG is performed intraoperatively, a triggered EMG threshold of 6.0 mA, coupled with threshold values of 60% to 65% decreased from the "average" of all other thresholds in a given patient, should be a red flag for scoliosis.

✦ In adult scoliosis unilateral radicular symptoms are much more common on the concavity side, and most symptoms are consistent with stenosis, with the notable exception that sitting does not relieve leg symptoms.

✦ In adult scoliosis the risk factors for curve progression include:
  – Cobb angle greater than 30 degrees
  – Apical rotation greater than grade II (Nash-Moe)
  – Lateral listhesis >6 mm
  – Intercrest line through or below L4-5 disc space

REFERENCES

1. Miller MD. Review of Orthopaedics, 3rd ed. Philadelphia: WB Saunders, 2000.
2. Lenke LG, Betz RR, Harms J. Modern Anterior Scoliosis Surgery. St Louis: Quality Medical Publishing, 2004.
3. Lenke LG, Edwards CC II, Bridwell KH. The Lenke classification of adolescent idiopathic scoliosis. How it organizes curve patterns as a template to perform selective fusions of the spine. Spine 28:S199-S207, 2003.
4. Whitaker C, Schoenecker PL, Lenke LG. Hyperkyphosis as an indicator of syringomyelia in idiopathic scoliosis: A case report. Spine 28:E16-E20, 2003.
5. Owen JH. The application of intraoperative monitoring during surgery for spinal deformity. Spine 24:2649-2662, 1999.
6. Raynor BL, Lenke LG, Kim Y, et al. Can triggered electromyograph thresholds predict safe thoracic pedicle screw placement? Spine 28:960, 2002.
7. Tribus CB. Scheuermann's kyphosis in adolescents and adults: Diagnosis and management. J Am Acad Orthop Surg 6:36-43, 1998.
8. O'Brien MF, Lenke LG, Mardjetko S, et al. Pedicle morphology in thoracic adolescent idiopathic scoliosis: Is pedicle fixation an anatomically viable technique? Spine 25:2285-2293, 2000.
9. Lenke LG, Betz RR, Harms J, et al. Adolescent idiopathic scoliosis: A new classification to determine extent of spinal arthrodesis. J Bone Joint Surg Am 83:1169-1181, 2001.
10. Lowe TG, Betz R, Lenke L, et al. Anterior single-rod instrumentation of the thoracic and lumbar spine: Saving levels. Spine 28:S208-S216, 2003.
11. Nash C, Moe J. A study of vertebral rotation. J Bone Joint Surg Am 51:223-229, 1969.
12. Sweet FA, Lenke LG, Bridwell KH, et al. Maintaining lumbar lordosis with anterior single solid-rod instrumentation in thoracolumbar and lumbar adolescent idiopathic scoliosis. Spine 24:1655-1662, 1999.

13. Vedantam R, Lenke LG, Bridwell KH, et al. A prospective evaluation of pulmonary function in patients with adolescent idiopathic scoliosis relative to the surgical approach used for spinal arthrodesis. Spine 25:82-90, 2000.

14. Paajanen H, Alanen A, Erkintalo M, et al. Disc degeneration in Scheuermann disease. Skeletal Radiol 18:523-526, 1989.

15. Sachs B, Bradford D, Winter R, et al. Scheuermann kyphosis. Follow-up of Milwaukee-brace treatment. J Bone Joint Surg Am 69:50-57, 1987.

16. Glassman SD, Rose SM, Dimar JR, et al. The effect of postoperative nonsteroidal anti-inflammatory drug administration on spinal fusion. Spine 23:834-838, 1998.

17. Herkowitz H. Surgical Options for "Discogenic" Low Back Pain. AAOS Instructional Course, 2002. Rosemont, IL: The Academy, 2002.

18. Spivak JM. Degenerative lumbar spinal stenosis. J Bone Joint Surg Am 80:1053-1066, 1998.

19. Tribus CB. Degenerative lumbar scoliosis evaluation and management. J Am Acad Orthop Surg 11:174-183, 2003.

20. Frishgrund J. Lumbar Degenerative Disorders of the Spine. Maine Review Course Lecture, 2003.

21. Lafage V, Schwab F, Vira S, et al. Spino-pelvic parameters after surgery can be predicted: A preliminary formula and validation of standing alignment. Spine 36:1037-1045, 2011.

22. Lafage V. Pelvic tilt and truncal inclination: Two key radiographic parameters in the setting of adults with spinal deformity. Spine 34:E599-E606, 2009.

23. Herkowitz HN, Sidhu KS. Lumbar spine fusion in the treatment of degenerative conditions: Current indication and recommendations. J Am Acad Orthop Surg 3:123-135, 1995.

24. McCord DH, Cunningham BW, Shono Y, et al. Biomechnical analysis of lumbosacral fixation. Spine 17(8 Suppl):S235-S243, 1992.

25. Kim JH, Horton W, Hamasaki T, et al. Spinal instrumentation for sacral-pelvic fixation: A biomechanical comparison between constructs ending with either S2 bicortical, bitriangulated screws or iliac screws. J Spinal Disord Tech 23:506-512, 2010.

26. Edwards CC, Bridwell KH, Patel A, et al. Long adult deformity fusions to L5 and the sacrum: A matched cohort analysis. Spine 29:1996-2005, 2004.

27. Tsuchiya K, Bridwell KH, Kuklo T, et al. Minimun 5-year analysis of L5-S1 fusion using sacropelvic fixation (bilateral S1 and iliac screws) for spinal deformity. Spine 31:303-308, 2006.

28. Kim YJ, Bridwell KH, Lenke LG, et al. Pseudarthrosis in adult spinal deformity following multisegmental instrumentation and arthrodesis. J Bone Joint Surg Am 88:721-728, 2006.

29. Tis JE, Helgeson M, Lehman R, et al. A biomechanical comparison of different types of lumbopelvic fixation. Spine 34:E866-E872, 2009.

30. O'Brien JR, Yu W, Bhatnagar R, et al. An anatomic study of the S2 iliac technique for lumbopelvic screw placement. Spine 34:E439-E442, 2009.

31. Chang TL, Sponseller PD, Kebaish KM, et al. Low profile pelvic fixation: Anatomic parameters for sacral alar-iliac fixation versus traditional iliac fixation. Spine 34:436-440, 2009.

32. O'Brien JR, Yu W, Kaufman BE, et al. Biomechanical evaluation of S2 alar-iliac screws: Effect of length and quad-cortical purchase as compared with iliac fixation. Spine 38:E1250-E1255, 2013.

33. Martin CT, Witham TF, Kebaish KM. Sacropelvic fixation: Two case reports of a new percutaneous technique. Spine 36:E618-E621, 2011.

7 ▪ Lumbar Radiculopathy

Lumbar radicular pain is defined as pain that originates in the lumbar spine and radiates from the lower back distally into one or both lower extremities. It is typically caused by disc or bony tissue compressing the nerve root. Such symptoms may also be produced by chemical irritation of the nerve root (or roots) by displaced disc tissue. The pain generally follows the dermatomal distribution of the affected nerve root.

SIGNS AND SYMPTOMS

- Radiculopathy usually presents with intermittent back pain before the onset of radiculopathy.[1]
- Radiculopathy can be mechanical pain (meaning relieved by rest) secondary to anular degeneration and is not always associated with trauma.
- Pain usually lessens in the lower back and becomes persistent in the leg.[1] Radicular pain is typically defined as radiating below the knee. Pain when sitting may be worse than when standing.
- Always be alert to cauda equina syndrome from a herniated disc, which is usually secondary to a large midline disc herniation at the lower lumbar levels L4-5 and L5-S1.
- Back and perianal pain usually predominates; saddle dysesthesias and radicular pain are minor and often bilateral.[1]
- 75% of patients experiencing bowel and bladder incontinence will regain function

> **Red Flag:** It is recommended that the patient be decompressed within the first 48 hours after onset of symptoms.[1] After that time, the potential for recovery is significantly worse.

> **Red Flag:** Be aware of painless weakness because it could be indicative of a tumor or infection.[1]

CLINICAL EVALUATION
Physical Examination

- Sensory dysesthesia follows dermatomal distribution. Nerve roots are mobile (i.e., L5 and S1 nerve roots can move from 2 to 6 mm, and herniations can affect them differently[1]; see ASIA examination on pp. 50 and 51).
- Straight leg raise is often more positive in younger patients than in older patients. Straight leg raise is considered positive if leg symptoms reproduced below the knee.
- Crossed straight leg raise has a high correlation with herniation, and reversed straight leg raise can be associated with high lumbar disc herniation.[1]

> **Red Flag:** Always be sure to check the vascular examination results as well as the range of motion of the hip and knee. Hip and knee pathology can also present similar to radicular complaints.

WORKUP
Radiographs

- Anteroposterior and lateral
- Flexion and extension

MRI

- One of the most helpful tests for identifying disc herniation that causes radicular pain.
- Sagittal and axial views should be reviewed with respect to the patient's presenting symptoms to better determine whether the imaged abnormality is related to the pain.

CT/Myelography

- CT/myelography may be helpful to further delineate the location and extent of neural compression

TREATMENT
Nonsurgical

- Physical therapy
- NSAIDs
- Medrol dose pack
- Antiinflammatory drugs
- Muscle relaxants
- Pain medications
- Selective nerve root block
  - Transforaminal epidural steroid injections (TFESIs)
    - It is questionable whether traditional epidural injections (both caudal and intralaminar types) deliver adequate concentrations of medication to target tissues.[2,3]
    - 84% of patients given TFESIs had successful outcomes over the follow-up period of 1.4 years (these results were obtained with an average of 1.7 injections as opposed to the traditionally prescribed 3 to 4 injections).[2,3]
    - Four mechanisms of action are in place to explain the high efficacy of TFESIs.[2,3]
      1. Precise delivery of steroid and xylocaine solution
      2. Nerve membrane-stabilizing properties of both the steroid and xylocaine

3. "Washout" effect of the solution, which decreases the regional levels of inflammation mediators
4. Potent antiinflammatory properties of the steroid

Surgical

- Indications
  - A minimum of 6 weeks of nonoperative care that does not resolve symptoms[1]
  - The patient presents with a progressive deficit, intractable pain, or cauda equina syndrome[1]
- See Intraoperative Management, Chapter 1, p. 2.
- Techniques
  - Laminotomy on the same side as the herniation
  - Bilateral laminotomy
  - Laminectomy
  - Endoscopic microdiscectomy
  - Chymopapain injection
    - ▸ Has recently received more attention and there is some thought to bringing this treatment back
    - ▸ Chymopapain splits the glycosaminoglycan side chain off from proteoglycan and decreases the ability of the nucleus to hold water[1]

Red Flag: Because of past complications, patients need to undergo pretesting to identify any sensitivity to papaya (chymopapain is derived from papaya).

Red Flag: Physicians and patients should be aware that there is a high incidence of postoperative low back pain with the chymopapain procedure.

- Complications
  - Anomalous nerve roots (double roots)
  - Disc herniations in the axilla of the nerve root
  - Synovial cysts: Can make the dura thin and more susceptible to tearing
    - ▸ Management of dural tears
      - ◆ Place the patient in reverse Trendelenburg position and attempt a watertight closure. Fibrin glue can be used or synthetic dura patches if the tear cannot be repaired. A drain is placed to gravity suction only and should not be removed until the patient is ambulatory. Antibiotics should be continued until the drain is removed. The patient should be on bed rest for a minimum of 24 hours. If the tear cannot be repaired, the patient should be placed on bed rest for 5 days. If fluid continues to leak out of the wound, options are to return to surgery or place a subarachnoid drain. The drain is placed by a surgeon or anesthesiologist in the operating room. The subarachnoid drain is raised or lowered until drainage is 10 to 20 cc/hr.

Red Flag: There is an increased risk of infection if cerebrospinal fluid is leaking from the wound.

  - Recurrent radicular pain[1]
    - ▸ Early (0-6 weeks): Think inadequate decompression, postoperative hematoma, infection[1]
    - ▸ Mid (6 weeks to 6 months): Think recurrent disc herniation, arachnoiditis, or pars fracture[1]
    - ▸ Late (>6 months): Think recurrent disc herniation, stenosis, or late instability[1]

PREDICTORS OF SURGICAL SUCCESS

If the following three predictors are positive, there is a 95% success rate; if two are positive one can expect an 85% success rate; and if one is positive, one can expect a 55% success rate[1]:

1. Positive imaging study
2. Positive straight leg raise
3. Neurologic deficit

KEY POINTS

✦ It is recommended that the patient be decompressed within the first 48 hours after the onset of symptoms. After that time, the potential for recovery is significantly worse.

✦ Be aware of painless weakness because it could be indicative of a tumor or infection.

✦ During the physical examination, always be sure to check both the vascular examination results and range of motion of the hip and knee. Hip and knee pathology can also present similar to radicular complaints.

✦ Because of past complications, patients need to undergo pretesting to identify any sensitivity to papaya (chymopapain is derived from papaya).

✦ Physicians and patients should be aware that there is a high incidence of postoperative low back pain with the chymopapain procedure.

✦ There is an increased risk of infection if cerebrospinal fluid is leaking from the wound.

REFERENCES

1. Frishgrund J. Lumbar Degenerative Disorders of the Spine. Maine Review Course Lecture, 2003.
2. Vad VB, Bhat AL, Lutz GE, et al. Transforaminal epidural steroid injections in lumbosacral radiculopathy: A prospective randomized study. Spine 27:11-16, 2002.
3. Riew KD, Yin Y, Gilula L, et al. Can nerve root injections obviate the need for operative treatment of lumbar radicular pain? A prospective, randomized, controlled, double-blind study. In Proceedings of the North American Spine Society, Fourteenth Annual Meeting, Chicago, 1999, pp 94-95.

8 ▪ Compression Fractures and Osteoporosis

Camden Whitaker and Ryan M. Stuckey

Bone strength is a combination of both bone mineral density (BMD) and the microarchitecture of bone. A decrease in BMD and/or a change in the microarchitecture can lead to osteoporotic fragility fractures. Hip fractures have an associated excess mortality rate of 8.4% to 36% at 1 year, and the mortality rate is higher in men than in women. In addition, the occurrence of a hip fracture increases the risk of a future fracture by 2.5 times. The presence of a single vertebral body compression fracture increases the risk of subsequent vertebral fractures fivefold and nonspine fragility fractures twofold to threefold.[1]

If a woman has two or more osteoporotic compression fractures, her risk of another fracture occurring is increased 12 times. A decrease of two standard deviations in BMD increases the risk 4 to 6 times; a positive family history increases the risk 2.7 times; premature menopause increases the risk 1.6 times; and smoking increases the risk 1.2 times.[2-4]

Type I primary osteoporosis generally occurs in women and begins 3 to 8 years after menopause as a result of estrogen deficiency. Type II primary osteoporosis typically occurs after the age of 70, and affects men and women. More than 50% of patients with osteoporosis will sustain some form of fracture, of which vertebral compression fractures are the most common.[5]

SIGNS AND SYMPTOMS

- Back pain, often with sudden, acute onset.
- Patient has a history of a previous fractured vertebra or has been treated with kyphoplasty and/or vertebroplasty or has an increased risk of compression fracture and/or osteoporosis.

CLINICAL EVALUATION
Risk Assessment

The initial diagnosis of osteoporosis begins with a risk assessment.

- All postmenopausal women and men ≥50 years old should be evaluated for the risk of osteoporosis. The risk assessment can then help determine which individuals require further testing with dual-energy X-ray absorptiometry (DEXA) and/or vertebral imaging and treatment.[6]
- The World Health Organization (WHO) has developed a fracture risk assessment tool known as FRAX, which calculates a 10-year absolute fracture risk.[7] The current variables in the FRAX model include:
  - Current age
  - Sex
  - Any previous osteoporotic fractures, including asymptomatic and clinical vertebral fractures
  - Femoral neck BMD (DEXA)
  - Rheumatoid arthritis
  - Low body mass index (kg/m^2)
  - Current smoker
  - Alcohol intake ≥3 drinks/day
  - Parental history of hip fracture
  - Oral glucocorticoids ≥5 mg/day of prednisone for ≥3 months (at any time)
  - Secondary osteoporosis
    - Insulin-dependent diabetes
    - Adults with osteogenesis imperfecta

- ▸ Long-standing untreated hyperthyroidism
- ▸ Hypogonadism
- ▸ Premature menopause (<45 years of age)
- ▸ Chronic malnutrition or malabsorption
- ▸ Chronic liver disease

Determining the Painful Level[8]

- Three-beat palpation to find pain correlates to the fractured compressed level.
  - Positive when palpation on the same spinal area three times reproduces pain.
- Edema on MRI
- Documentation of recent fracture

WORKUP

- Routine radiographs
  - The National Osteoporosis Foundation (NOF) has developed recommendations for vertebral imaging. Vertebral imaging (assessment of lateral vertebral fractures by DEXA or conventional radiographs) is recommended for the following patients[6]:
    - ▸ All women ≥70 years old and men ≥80 years old
    - ▸ In women ages 65 to 69 with a BMD T-score ≤1.5
    - ▸ Postmenopausal women ages 50 to 64 and men ages 50 to 59 with risk factors including:
      - ◆ Low trauma fracture
      - ◆ Height loss of ≥1.5 inches (4 cm)
      - ◆ Recent or ongoing long-term glucocorticoid treatment
- MRI
  - Presence of edema
  - Hemangioma on MRI[2]
    - ▸ Large hemangiomas have vertical striations and may be visible on plain radiographs.

- ▸ Axial CT scans commonly reveal a speckled appearance.
- ▸ Metastatic lesions are typically hypointense on T1-weighted images because they replace the fatty marrow.
- ▸ Bony islands, like cortical bone, are dark on T1- and T2-weighted images.
- Bone Mineral Density
  - According to the NOF's *Clinician's Guide to Prevention and Treatment of Osteoporosis*,[1] BMD testing should be considered for the following patients:
    - ▸ Women ≥65 years of age and men ≥70 years of age
    - ▸ Younger postmenopausal women, women in menopausal transition, and men ages 50 to 69 with clinical risk factors for a fracture
    - ▸ Adults who sustain a fracture after age 50
    - ▸ Adults with a condition or taking a medication associated with decreased bone mass or bone loss (e.g., glucocorticoids ≥5 mg of prednisone or the equivalent for ≥3 months)
  - BMD is evaluated with a DEXA scan. DEXA scan results are reported as T-scores and Z-scores.
    - ▸ T-score: The number of standard deviations a patient's BMD is above or below the peak BMD for an average 30 year old of the same sex and race.
    - ▸ WHO defines osteopenia as a T-score between −1 and −2.5. Osteoporosis is defined as a T-score ≤2.5.
    - ▸ Z-score: The number of standard deviations a patient's BMD is above or below the expected peak BMD for someone of the same age, sex, and race.
  - The history or presence of a vertebral body fracture is consistent with the diagnosis of osteoporosis, even if the BMD is nondiagnostic for osteoporosis. This diagnosis alone is an indication for treatment with an osteoporosis medication.

- ▸ Treatment should be considered in postmenopausal women and in men ages 50 and older who have any of the following[1,6]:
  - ◆ T-score of ≤−2.5 measured at the femoral neck, total hip, or lumbar spine
  - ◆ T-score −1.0 and −2.5 and a 10-year probability of a hip fracture ≥3% or a 10-year probability of a major osteoporosis-related fracture ≥20% based on the U.S.-adapted WHO osteoporosis algorithm (FRAX)
  - ◆ Any hip or vertebral fracture, independent of the T-score

TREATMENT/MANAGEMENT
Medical/Pharmacologic Management

- ▪ The medical management of osteoporosis starts with optimizing the daily intake of calcium and vitamin D (Table 8-1).
- ▪ Pharmacologic management of osteoporosis is divided into antiresorptive agents and anabolic agents.
  - • The antiresorptive agents include bisphosphonates (Table 8-2), estrogen/hormone replacement therapy (Table 8-3), selective estrogen receptor modulators (SERMs) (Table 8-3), receptor activator of nuclear factor kappa-B ligand (RANKL) inhibitor (Table 8-4), and calcitonin (Table 8-5).[1,9-11]
  - • The only anabolic agent currently available for the treatment of postmenopausal osteoporosis is teriparatide (Forteo) (rhPTH[1-34]; Table 8-6).[1,9-11]

Table 8-1 Recommended Daily Intake of Calcium and Vitamin D

	Recommended Daily Calcium Intake (mg)	Recommended Daily Vitamin D Intake (IU)
Patient age (yr)		
<50	1000	1000
>50	1200	1000
Fracture healing	1500-2500	1000-2000

Text continued on p. 170.

Table 8-2   Bisphosphonates Antiresorptive Agents[1,9-11]

Generic Name	Trade Name	Approved Indications	Recommended Dosing
Alendronate	Fosamax	Prevention and treatment of osteoporosis in postmenopausal women and men Treatment of osteoporosis in patients taking glucocorticoids	5 mg po daily or 35 mg po weekly (prevention) 10 mg po daily or 70 mg po weekly (treatment)
Ibandronate	Boniva	Treatment of postmenopausal osteoporosis	150 mg po monthly 3 mg IV q 3 mo
Risedronate	Actonel	Prevention and treatment of osteoporosis in postmenopausal women and men and treatment of osteoporosis in patients taking glucocorticoids	5 mg po daily or 35 mg po weekly 75 mg po for 2 consecutive days/mo 150 mg po monthly
Zoledronate	Reclast	Prevention and treatment of osteoporosis in postmenopausal women and men Treatment of osteoporosis in patients taking glucocorticoids or expected to be taking glucocorticoids for 12 mo Prevention of new clinical fractures in patients with recent low trauma hip fracture	5 mg IV infusion/yr (treatment) 5 mg IV infusion/2 yr (prevention)

Cr Cl, Creatinine clearance; *GFR,* glomerular filtration rate; *VBC,* vertebral body compression.

Table 8-3   Estrogen Agonist/Antagonists or SERMs Antiresorptive Agents[1,9-11]

Generic Name	Trade Name	Approved Indications	Recommended Dosing
Raloxifene	Evista	Prevention and treatment of osteoporosis in postmenopausal women	60 mg po daily

DVT, Deep vein thrombosis; *SERMs,* selective estrogen receptor modulators; *VBC,* vertebral body compression.

Efficacy	Adverse Effects	Contraindications
Reduces incidence of spine and hip fractures by 50% over 3 yr in patients with previous VBC fractures and by 48% in patients without a previous VBC fracture	Esophageal inflammation, gastric ulcer, osteonecrosis of the jaw, atypical subtrochanteric and diaphyseal femoral fractures	Severe renal insufficiency (GFR <30-35 ml/min), esophageal motility problems, hypocalcemia, inability to sit or stand upright for 30 min
Reduces incidence of VBC fractures 50% over 3 yr	Same as above	Same as above
Reduces incidence of VBC fractures 41%-49% over 3 yr and nonvertebral fractures 36% over 3 yr	Same as above	Same as above
Reduces incidence of VBC fractures 70%, hip fractures 41%, and nonvertebral fractures by 25% over 3 yr	Same as above	Cr Cl <35 ml/min (Cr Cl should be monitored before every dose of zoledronate)

Efficacy	Adverse Effects	Contraindications
Reduces risk of VBC fractures by 30% in patients with a prior VBC fracture and 55% in patients without a prior VBC fracture over 3 yr. Reduction in risk of nonvertebral fracture with raloxifene has not been documented	Increases risk of DVT	Premenopausal women and in women with a history of DVT or other thromboembolic events

Table 8-4 Receptor Activator of Nuclear Factor kappa-B (RANK) Ligand (RANKL)/RANKL Inhibitor[1,9-11]

Generic Name	Trade Name	Approved Indications	Recommended Dosing
Denosumab	Prolia	Treatment of osteoporosis in post-menopausal women at high risk of a fracture Increase bone mass in men at high risk of a fracture Treatment of bone loss in women with breast cancer Treatment of bone loss in men undergoing certain treatments for prostate cancer	60 mg SQ q 6 mo by a health care professional

VBC, Vertebral body compression.

Table 8-5 Calcitonin Antiresorptive Agent[1,9-11]

Generic Name	Trade Name	Approved Indications	Recommended Dosing
Calcitonin	Miacalcin or Fortical	Treatment for women >5 yr postmenopausal	200 IU/day by intranasal spray

VBC, Vertebral body compression.

Table 8-6 Parathyroid Hormone [rhPTH(1-34)] Anabolic Agent[1,9-11]

Generic Name	Trade Name	Approved Indications	Recommended Dosing
Teriparatide	Forteo	Treatment of osteoporosis in postmenopausal women at high risk of a fracture Treatment of osteoporosis in patients taking glucocorticoids Increase bone mass in men with primary or hypogonadal osteoporosis	20 mg daily SQ injection

VBC, Vertebral body compression.

Efficacy	Adverse Effects	Contraindications
Reduces incidence of VBC fractures by 68%, hip fractures 40%, and nonvertebral fractures 20% over 3 yr	Hypocalcemia, increased risk of skin infection and rash, osteonecrosis of the jaw, atypical femur fractures Stopping denosumab treatment can cause rapid bone loss; alternative treatment should be considered to maintain BMD	Hypocalcemia

Efficacy	Adverse Effects	Contraindications
Reduces incidence of VBC fractures by 30% in patients with previous VBC fractures, but has not been shown to reduce nonvertebral fractures	Rhinitis, epistaxis, allergic reaction in patients allergic to salmon	Patients with salmon allergies

Efficacy	Adverse Effects	Contraindications
Reduces risk of VBC fractures by 65% and nonvertebral fractures by 53% in patients with osteoporosis after 18 mo of treatment	Increased risk of osteosarcoma (seen in rat trials; no documented cases in humans treated for 18 mo and followed for >3 yr) Leg cramps, nausea, dizziness	Paget disease, increased risk of osteosarcoma, previous radiation therapy, bone metastases, history of skeletal malignant tumors, hypercalcemia

Nonsurgical

- Bracing
- NSAIDs
- Physical therapy
- Pain medication

Surgical

- General indications[8]
  - No improvement after 6 weeks of nonoperative treatment
  - No infectious or oncologic etiologic factors
- Early surgical intervention considerations[8]
  - Potential for collapse T11-L2
  - Stable burst pattern; in elderly (not high energy) patients, no retropulsion
  - >30 degrees of kyphosis
  - Progressive collapse
  - Hospital admission for pain control
- Techniques
  - Kyphoplasty[4] (Fig. 8-1, pp. 171-174)
    - ▸ Vertebral augmentation by kyphoplasty, according to the early studies, is clearly an effective treatment for painful, progressive, osteoporotic compression fractures.
    - ▸ Kyphoplasty minimizes the risk of cement leakage by compacting the cancellous bone to the periphery and sealing off the fracture clefts and by creating a cavity into which cement is poured, as opposed to injected under pressure.
    - ▸ This technique may prevent propagation of further fractures by reducing the collapsed vertebral bodies toward their native height, thus normalizing the sagittal spinal alignment.
    - ▸ Indications
      - ◆ <3 months postfracture.
      - ◆ Osteoporotic bone.
      - ◆ Edema on MRI.

Text continued on p. 175.

TRANSPEDICULAR APPROACH

Fig. 8-1 Kyphoplasty. (From Inflatable Bone Tamp Technology Course. Memphis, TN: Kyphon, Sept 2003. KYPHON® Balloon Kyphoplasty incorporates technology developed by Gary K. Michelson, MD.)   *Continued*

TRANSPEDICULAR APPROACH

Final position

Midpedicle too medial

Too far medial

Too far lateral

Fig. 8-1, cont'd Kyphoplasty. (From Inflatable Bone Tamp Technology Course. Memphis, TN: Kyphon, Sept 2003. KYPHON® Balloon Kyphoplasty incorporates technology developed by Gary K. Michelson, MD.)

EXTRAPEDICULAR APPROACH

Midpedicle

Posterior vertebral body wall

Midbody position

Fig. 8-1, cont'd Kyphoplasty. (From Inflatable Bone Tamp Technology Course. Memphis, TN: Kyphon, Sept 2003. KYPHON® Balloon Kyphoplasty incorporates technology developed by Gary K. Michelson, MD.) *Continued*

EXTRAPEDICULAR APPROACH

Final position

Too far medial

Too far lateral

Fig. 8-1, cont'd Kyphoplasty. (From Inflatable Bone Tamp Technology Course. Memphis, TN: Kyphon, Sept 2003. KYPHON® Balloon Kyphoplasty incorporates technology developed by Gary K. Michelson, MD.)

- ◆ Progressive collapse.
- ◆ The greater the edema or signal intensity, the better the reduction potential.
- ◆ If, after a 6-week trial of nonsurgical management, progressive collapse of the vertebral body is shown on radiographs, the patient's pain is incapacitating and/or difficult to control, or the patient requires hospitalization or does not respond to conservative care, kyphoplasty can be recommended.[4]
  - ▸ The ideal timing for a kyphoplasty procedure is controversial. Acute vertebral compression fractures (VCF) and minor degrees of vertebral collapse can be followed closely with serial radiographs for a 6-week trial.[4]
    - ◆ Special circumstances that can cause vertebrae to collapse are thoracolumbar junction fractures, fractures caused by steroid-induced osteoporosis, or fractures that have occurred in vertebrae with extremely low bone mineral density.[4] These deformities can be treated earlier with kyphoplasty.
  - ▸ If advanced sagittal plane malalignment or kyphosis already exists at presentation, kyphoplasty should be considered immediately to improve sagittal alignment.
- Vertebroplasty[12]
  - ▸ The most common use of vertebroplasty is to treat vertebral fractures resulting from osteoporosis.
  - ▸ In vertebral compression fractures related to osteoporosis, the beneficial effect of percutaneous vertebroplasty to relieve pain is favorable.
  - ▸ The percutaneous vertebroplasty procedure is timely, because there has been a great need for rapid and effective therapy, particularly in the osteoporotic patient population.
  - ▸ Indications for vertebroplasty with cavitation.
    - ◆ More than 3 months postfracture
    - ◆ Nonosteoporotic bone

- No edema on MRI
- Healed fractures
- No progressive collapse
- Pseudarthrosis, fibrous: Fibrous union
‣ Management of complications of vertebroplasty[4,13]
  - Extravertebral cement extravasation can occur during vertebroplasty, with leak rates of up to 65%.
  - An increased rate of extravasation has been demonstrated in patients with tumors (metastases or hemangiomas) compared with patients with osteoporosis.
  - To decrease the risk of extravertebral cement leakage, intravertebral contrast injection studies have been recommended before cement injection to predict the extrusion of cement.
  - McGraw et al[13] found that intraosseus venography predicted the subsequent flow of bone cement during vertebroplasty in 83% of cases.
  - Gaughen et al reported that during vertebroplasty, 22 (52%) treated vertebrae demonstrated cement extravasation, and in 14 of these 22 cases they noted venous involvement with venograms demonstrating extravasation.
▪ Contraindications/precautions for vertebroplasty and kyphoplasty procedures
  • Patient factors
    ‣ Young age
    ‣ Sepsis
    ‣ Cardiopulmonary compromise
    ‣ Bleeding disorders or anticoagulation therapy
  • Fracture factors
    ‣ High-energy injury.
    ‣ Significant burst component.

- ▸ Neurologic compromise related to fracture.
- ▸ Posterior vertebral body wall deficiency or fracture.
- ▸ Fracture limits access to the vertebral body (i.e., pedicle fracture or pedicle compromise).
- ▸ Surgeon unable to visualize the fracture with intraoperative radiography/fluoroscopy.
- ▸ Unstable sagittal balance.
- ▸ Vertebra plana.

- More than three vertebral levels during one operative setting, because deleterious cardiopulmonary effects related to cement and/or fat embolization to the lungs have been reported.
- Disc degeneration, internal disc disruption, or Schmorl's nodes limit the ability to fully control the pain generator. In these patients with discogenic pain, fusion may be a more appropriate option.
- Levels superior to T5 are difficult to visualize.
- Extension injuries: If the injury involves the posterior element structures and the anterior vertebral body is not collapsed, this is a contraindication to surgery.
- Disc involvement: If there is an infection present, this is a contraindication to surgery.
- Kummell's disease: A vacuum cleft on an anteroposterior radiograph can be a sign of avascular necrosis of the vertebral body and can be difficult to heal.[4,14]
- Chronic osteoporotic compression fractures are usually not associated with MRI signal changes. In contrast, a low signal intensity on T1-weighted images and high signal intensity on T2-weighted images can be seen with avascular necrosis.[4,14] Maldague et al[14] were the first to describe this phenomenon. The majority of these patients were immunosuppressed: 7 of 10 patients were receiving long-term systemic steroid therapy, one

had radiation therapy, and one had cirrhosis. Kummell's disease is pathognomonic for avascular necrosis.[14] Also, vertebral body collapse and gas dissecting into adjacent psoas musculature suggests avascular necrosis.[14] Interestingly, the vacuum cleft can disappear in flexion.[14]

- Tumors[8]
- Fractures superior to T6

> **Red Flag:** Compression fractures in males are rare. Perform additional testing to ensure that it is a compression fracture and that a tumor is not present.

- Pedicle or soft tissue extension
- If the tumor has caused posterior vertebral body or neural element involvement
- Open surgery for kyphoplasty and vertebroplasty
  - Open surgery rather than percutaneous surgery is indicated for patients with severe, painful, rigid sagittal deformities that significantly limit the patient's quality of life and function.[3]

Postoperative Considerations

- Physical therapy to help with the muscle injury or pain associated with fracture[5]

KEY POINTS

✦ If a woman has two or more osteoporotic compression fractures, her risk of another fracture occurring is increased 12 times.

✦ Compression fractures in men are rare. Additional testing should be performed to ensure that it is a compression fracture and that a tumor is not present.

✦ The presence of a single vertebral body compression fracture increases the risk of subsequent vertebral fractures fivefold and non-spine fragility fractures two- to threefold.

✦ If advanced sagittal plane malalignment or kyphosis already exists at presentation, kyphoplasty should be considered immediately to improve sagittal alignment.

✦ In vertebral compression fractures related to osteoporosis, the beneficial effect of percutaneous vertebroplasty to relieve pain is favorable.

REFERENCES

1. National Osteoporosis Foundation. Clinician's Guide to Prevention and Treatment of Osteoporosis. Washington, DC: National Osteoporosis Foundation, 2013.
2. American Academy of Orthopaedic Surgeons. Orthopaedic Special Interest Examination 2003. Adult Spine Self-Assessment Examination.
3. Melton LJ III. Epidemiology of spinal osteoporosis. Spine 22(24 Suppl):S2-S11, 1997.
4. Phillips FM. Minimally invasive treatments of osteoporotic vertebral compression fractures. Spine 28(15 Suppl):S45-S53, 2003.
5. Togawa D, Leiberman IH. Pain, biomechanics, and thoracic restoration technique. In Maxwell JH, Griffith SL, Welch WC, eds. Nonfusion Techniques for the Spine: Motion Preservation and Balance. St Louis: Quality Medical Publishing, 2006.
6. Dell RM, Greene D, Anderson D, et al. Osteoporosis disease management: What every orthopaedic surgeon should know. J Bone Joint Surg Am 91 (Suppl 6):79-86, 2009.
7. FRAX calculator. Available at *http://www.shef.ac.uk/FRAX/*
8. Kyphon Instructional Course: Images from the Inflatable Bone Tamp Technology Course. Memphis, TN: Kyphon, Sept 2003.
9. Lehman R Jr, Dmitriev AE, Cardoso MJ, et al. Effect of teriparatide [rhPTH-(1-34)] and calcitonin on intertransverse process fusion in a rabbit model. Spine 35:146-152, 2010.
10. Ohtori S, Inoue G, Orita S, et al. Comparison of teriparatide and bisphosphonate treatment to reduce pedicle screw loosening after lumbar spinal fusion surgery in postmenopausal women with osteoporosis from a bone quality perspective. Spine 38:E487-E492, 2013.

11. Gehrig L, Lane J, O'Connor MI. Osteoporosis: Management and treatment strategies for orthopaedic surgeons. Instr Course Lect 58:817-832, 2009.
12. Kostuik J. Vertebral body augmentation: History, current technique, and future considerations. In Corbin TP, Connolly PJ, Yuan HA, et al, eds. Emerging Spine Surgery Technologies. Evidence and Framework for Evaluating New Technology. St Louis: Quality Medical Publishing, 2006.
13. McGraw JK, Heatwole EV, Strnad BT, et al. Predictive value of intraosseous venography before percutaneous vertebroplasty. J Vasc Interv Radiol 13 (2 Pt 1):149-153, 2002.
14. Maldague BE, Noel HM, Malghem J. The intravertebral vacuum cleft: A sign of ischemic vertebral collapse. Radiology 129:23-29, 1978.

9 ▪ Low Back Pain

Camden Whitaker and Ryan M. Stuckey

One of the most difficult tasks in treating patients with low back pain is narrowing the differential or defining the patient's problems. Before beginning treatment, whether operative or nonoperative, determining the pain generator is essential. A complete history and physical examination are mandatory, as is defining exacerbating activities, and pain at rest or during activity, as well as psychosocial issues and issues of secondary gain.[1] The latter two can confound both the diagnosis and treatment.

DEFINING THE PROBLEM: CAUSES OF LOW BACK PAIN[2]
Discogenic Low Back Pain

- Characterized by axial pain originating from an inflammatory area in the disc anulus.
- Can be caused by an anular tear, previous surgery, instability, degenerative disc disease, or internal disc disruption.

Degenerative Disc Disease

- May result from age-related arthritic changes that are usually painless.
- Radiographic results show disc space narrowing, sclerosis of endplates, osteophyte formation, and retrolisthesis.

Internal Disc Derangement

- A normal-appearing disc may have pain originating from an anular injury.

Anular Tear

- An outer-edge anular disruption that may be associated with an audible "pop."
- An anular tear can result from acute low back pain that does not improve.
- MRI can confirm the diagnosis; many anular tears can be painless.

High-Intensity Zone

- The high-intensity zone (HIZ) is identified as a small, round lesion that shows a bright signal along the posterior-inferior anulus on T2-weighted images. These lesions are associated with an anular tear in more than 90% of cases with discography.

Endplate or Modic Changes

- Changes in bone marrow seen on MRI show a signal (bright on T2-weighted images, dark on T1-weighted images) adjacent to the vertebral endplate. They often correspond to sclerosis on plain radiographs.
- Significance is controversial.

Instability

- Instability is poorly defined.
- Definition: For chronic low back pain, a minimum of 5 mm anteroposterior motion or 11 degrees of flexion-extension angulation.
- Isthmic defects with >4 mm of spondylolisthesis should be considered "unstable," since they are likely to be a cause of chronic low back pain.

Chronic Low Back Pain

- Low back pain is defined as chronic if daily symptoms that interfere with quality of life have persisted for more than 6 months.

SIGNS AND SYMPTOMS

Diagnosis is often difficult because many pain generators refer pain to similar areas or regions. One always has to be on the lookout for inconsistencies of examination findings and nonanatomic complaints, which might suggest a nonorganic pain component.[1] The problem must be defined by separating back pain from leg pain. Leg pain may start and stay in the buttocks and present with paresthesias in the distal extremity. Patients frequently present without dynamic films, and spondylolisthesis is often missed with static films.[1] Obtaining flexion and extension radiographs is essential to rule out the diagnosis of dynamic spondylolisthesis. Standing and dynamic MRI might provide a better understanding of this diagnosis. It is helpful to classify low back pain into the following six categories.

1. Neurogenic
2. Spondylogenic
3. Inflammatory/arthritic
4. Neoplastic
5. Discogenic
6. Soft tissue

Waddell Criteria

- Waddell noted that most patients with documented organic low back pain had one or none of the Waddell criteria, and that patients who had three of five Waddell criteria were much more likely to have nonorganic low back pain.[3]
- Waddell's five criteria/findings on physical examination that correlate with nonorganic low back pain[2]
    1. Tenderness: Superficial (light pinch), nonanatomic (tender to palpation over lumbar spine, pelvis, and thoracic spine).
    2. Pain on simulated rotation: Axial loading (should not cause low back pain) and pelvic rotation.

3. Distraction: Straight-leg raise is painless with distraction.
4. Regional: Give-way weakness, sensory loss (nonanatomic distribution).
5. Overreaction (most important): Patient responds inappropriately to light touch.

Red Flag: Watch out for the following[4]: (1) Waddell's sign; (2) low back pain after discectomy—consider discitis, which is extremely painful; (3) history of neoplasm; (4) excessive morning stiffness (especially when associated with other inflammatory joints); and (5) night pain, fever, chills, and weight loss.

CLINICAL EVALUATION

- Obtain complete history and perform thorough physical examination.
- Define exacerbating activities and pain at rest or during activity.
- Be aware that psychosocial issues are of secondary gain.
- Determine the patient's treatment course to date.
- Perform a neurologic examination, grading the patient's strength, sensation, reflexes, bowel or bladder changes, and sexual function.
- Define the pain generator; examining the patient during flexion and extension might provide clues. Extension may exacerbate facet arthrosis, whereas flexion can exacerbate disc disorders.
- Palpate for tenderness along the facet joints.
- Test the sacroiliac joint to aid in the diagnosis.
  - Perform the flexion-abduction external rotation (FABER) test to evaluate, or the finger-point test to assess the sacroiliac joint.
- Test nerve tension by having the patient perform straight-leg raises in the supine or sitting position.
- Test the posterior nerves as well as the femoral nerves.

WORKUP
Plain Radiographs

- Source of pain can be nonspecific.[5]
- Usually not indicated for the first 6 weeks of acute low back pain because the pain will resolve in 90% of cases.
- In patients 50 years of age and older, radiographs may lack correlation between pain and degenerative changes seen on the film.[6]
- Radiographic findings to look for: Isolated disc space narrowing, especially L5-S1; pars defects; spondylolisthesis; retrolisthesis; lumbar mobile segments; transitional levels; lateral listhesis; intact pedicles; scoliosis; spina bifida; and previous surgery (e.g., status post laminectomy).
- Dynamic radiographs should also be obtained; unfortunately, there is no standardized technique or definition of instability.[6]
  - The quality of the films can be limited by patient positioning or rotation. Painful instability is demonstrated with anterior-posterior translation of >5 mm, spondylolisthesis or retrolisthesis of >4 mm, or a pars defect.[6]

Technetium Bone Scan

- Can be used to assess pars defects.
- Has a low sensitivity and specificity, but SPECT imaging increases sensitivity for pars defects and other posterior element lesions.[6]

MRI

- Highly sensitive to degenerative changes.
- Determining which changes are painful can make interpretation of findings difficult.[5]
- Disc degeneration is most commonly seen at L4-5 and L5-S1.[6] A black disc on T2-weighted images correlates with disc degeneration, but as Boden et al[5] demonstrated, MRIs in asymptomatic people can show disc herniations in 25% and disc degeneration in 54%.

- Other MRI findings include hydration of discs, disc space narrowing, generalized wide-based disc bulge, focal disc herniations, foraminal narrowing, far-lateral disc herniations, endplate changes, retrolisthesis, Schmorl's nodes, and discitis in postdiscectomy patients.[6]
- Gadolinium is added to differentiate between scar and recurrent herniation.
- An MRI does not show lateral recess stenosis as well as a CT scan can.

Lumbar Discography (Table 9-1)

- Used to determine whether dark discs are painful and surrounding discs are painless.[6,7]
- Based on pressure, morphology, and pain concordance; symptoms that are difficult to interpret in people with psychological problems.[5]
- A CT scan is needed to check the position of the dye used in the discogram to evaluate the morphology.
- False positives can occur with anulus and endplate injections.
- It is important not to oversedate the patient during the discogram, because the patient must be able to verbalize his or her pain response.
- Can also be used if a patient presents complaining only of back pain and with an MRI scan that is difficult to interpret and in those who are worried about a recurrent herniated disc.
  - In this same situation, if the patient complains of leg pain, a CT myelogram would be more prudent.
- In difficult-to-interpret discography, xylocaine can be injected into a painful disc, because a painful disc can still be irritated from the disc injection above—a pressure phenomenon causing normal discs to appear painful during discography.
  - If the patient has an anular leak, the xylocaine can anesthetize the spine and complicate the results.
- If the patient is allergic to dye, gadolinium can be used.

Table 9-1 Discography Classifications

Disc Classification	Intradiscal Pressure at Pain Provocation	Pain Severity	Pain Type	Ruling
Chemical	Immediate onset of familiar pain occurring as <1 ml of contrast is visualized reaching the outer anulus,* or pain provocation at <15 psi (103.5 kPa) above opening pressure	≥6/10	Concordant	Positive
Mechanical	Between 15 and 50 psi (103.5 to 344.7 kPa) above opening pressure	≥6/10	Concordant	Positive (but other pain generators may be present; further investigation may be warranted)
Indeterminate	Between 51 and 90 psi (346.2 to 620.5 kPa)	≥6/10	Concordant	Further investigation warranted
Normal	>90 psi (620.5 kPa)	No pain		Negative

From Derby R, Howard MW, Grant JM, et al. The ability of pressure-controlled discography to predict surgical and nonsurgical outcomes. Spine 24:364-371, 1999.

*Typically the contrast medium will be visualized reaching the outer anulus at <10 psi above the opening pressure. Consequently a disc generating familiar concordant pain as contrast is visualized reaching the outer anulus may be deemed chemically sensitive as defined within the context of this study.

kPa, kPascal; *psi*, pounds per square inch.

- A painful disc leaks from the center either posteriorly toward the canal or peripherally in the anulus.[6]
- If more volume is required, a tear may be indicated because the normal volume of a lumbar disc is between 0.5 and 1.5 cc and between 0.1 and 0.3 cc in the cervical spine.
- Discography anatomy and pressure
  - Location of the tear is predictive[8]
    - 75% of patients with single-level anterior-posterior fusion at the L5-S1 level with outer anular tears (abnormal MRI) had a good outcome.
    - 50% with only inner tears (normal MRI) had a good outcome.

- Pressure stratification
  - ▸ Chemically sensitive disc: <15 PSI, dye leaking at anulus.[9]
  - ▸ Mechanically sensitive disc: >50 PSI.[9]
  - ▸ Results are better when chemically sensitive discs are treated with anterior interbody fusion.[9]
- Complications
  - Patients may have increased pain for 1 to 2 weeks after the procedure.

> **Red Flag:** More worrisome is the <1% risk of discitis, which has been shown to decrease with the use of the double-needle technique.[6]

- Long-term follow-up
  - Few animal studies that have been performed have demonstrated no long-term effects.
  - Johnson[10] reported no long-term effects in 34 patients who had a second discography.
  - Flanagan and Chung[4] found no significant changes in 188 patients 10 to 20 years after they had a normal discogram.
  - Discography remains controversial in certain areas of the country because of the findings of the Holt study.[6] This study contradicted the value of discography. In 30 asymptomatic prisoners with normal discs, Holt et al injected 72 discs (18 failures) using a 24-gauge needle with 1 to 2 cc 50% Hypaque material.[11] Holt reported 37% false positives. Many authors have criticized the Holt study, citing the following problems: The high failure rate, the fact that no fluoroscopy was used, the possibility of anular injections, injection of normal discs, needle accuracy, and use of a very irritating contrast medium.[6] Despite numerous studies validating the use of discography, many opponents still quote this study.
  - Concordant pain response: Colhoun et al[12] studied 137 patients with positive pain provocation and compared them with 25 pa-

tients who had abnormal morphology with no pain. All were treated with 360-degree fusions; 89% of the patients who had a positive pain response had a good outcome versus 52% of the patients who had no pain response and had a good outcome.[12]

TREATMENT/MANAGEMENT
Conservative Treatment

Conservative treatment for low back pain is not well defined because a large percentage of patients improve over time. Treatment has an increased chance of success when patients are active participants in their care. The best treatment combines patient education with rehabilitation.[1,13] There are many conservative treatment options and most are used in combination (for example, bed rest, medications, physical therapy, chiropractic care, injections, and bracing).

- Bed rest
  - Despite conflicting reports in the literature, bed rest is a common treatment for low back pain. Some authors have demonstrated that bed rest can provide a limited benefit for overall pain[13]; others have shown a quicker return to work with little or no bed rest.[14]
  - The general recommendation is for short-term bed rest (maximum of 2 days), if necessary.[1,14]
- Medications
  - Medications should be used as an adjunct to physical therapy; they should never be promoted as a cure and should be used judiciously because of numerous side effects.[1,6]
  - Medications include NSAIDs, steroids, muscle relaxants, analgesics, antidepressants, and antiseizure medications.
    - NSAIDs
      - Used for inflammatory conditions of the major joints of the body.
      - Their mechanism of action is through inhibition of prostaglandin synthesis and cyclooxygenase (COX) activity.[1]

- With the recent release of the COX-2 inhibitors, they have been promoted as having similar effects without the side effects. Almost 16,000 people a year die from gastrointestinal bleeding, and antiinflammatory drugs have been a major culprit.
- COX-1 inhibitors maintain cellular homeostasis, whereas COX-2 activity is induced by inflammatory mediators.[1] These medications can be used differently for different effects. For example, when the dosage is regular, they are used as antiinflammatory drugs but when the dosage is intermittent, they are used as analgesics.[1]

Red Flag: Pay attention to the warning on the Celebrex label.

- ▸ Steroids
  - Used to treat acute nerve root irritation resulting from herniated discs.
  - Administered in dose packs.
  - Play a minimal role in the treatment of low back pain.[1]
  - Side effects of steroids can be significant and include gastrointestinal bleeding, increased risk of infection, avascular necrosis, and osteopenia, if used over long periods of time. Wound healing can be affected as well.
- ▸ Muscle relaxants
  - Used for acute low back pain.
  - Some literature reports that muscle relaxants are more effective than placebo alone.[1]
- ▸ Analgesics
  - Includes opioids and acetaminophen. Opioids can be used to control acute pain but their use for chronic pain remains controversial—possibility of abuse and addiction.[1] Opioid side effects include drowsiness, dizziness, fatigue, nausea, respiratory depression, and constipation. If combined with

acetaminophen, an overdose of acetaminophen can lead to hepatic toxicity.[15,16]

- ◆ Short-acting narcotics can cause sleep deprivation (despite their use to help with sleep) and are more often abused.[1,15,16]
- ◆ Long-acting opioids are less addicting, better tolerated, and have fewer side effects.[1]
- ◆ Avoidance of all narcotics is best, if possible.[1,15,16] If narcotics are part of the patient's treatment, prepare a Narcotic Patient Contract outlining an appropriate refill schedule. Many pharmacies have computer systems that monitor doctor shopping, refill scheduling, and use of other pharmacies.

- ▸ Antidepressants and antiseizure medication
  - ◆ Associated mood disorders and psychosocial diagnoses are prevalent in patients with low back pain.
  - ◆ Depression can cause and/or exacerbate low back pain, and anxiety can lower one's pain threshold.[1]
  - ◆ A multispecialty approach is best.
  - ◆ Antiseizure medication is most effective when used along with other medical treatments.

- ■ Physical therapy
  - • Physical therapy is the mainstay of nonoperative treatment for low back pain.[1,5] Physical therapy has been shown to be more effective than medicine alone for low back pain over a 6-month time period.[3] Although some literature identifies equivalent success compared to chiropractic for acute pain, physical therapy is better than chiropractic for chronic pain. A medically guided and monitored physical therapy exercise program has been shown to be more successful than unsupervised exercises.[1,3]
  - • A physical therapy program should be designed with the goal of developing core strength or the muscular columns needed to support the spine. It is especially important to strengthen the multifundus. Directional training or exercising the patient in the least symptomatic direction is recommended—for example, pa-

tients should perform flexion exercises if they experience increased pain in extension.[1,6]

- The goal is to improve flexibility, trunk muscle strengthening, and posture.[5,17,18]
- The literature has reported that treatment consisting only of physical modalities (i.e., massage and ultrasound) provide limited benefits.[1]

- Chiropractic
  - The exact mechanism of chiropractic care in achieving pain relief is not clear.[1] It has been well established that for acute low back pain 5 to 10 treatments can be beneficial. Chiropractic care is more effective than medical care alone and is as effective as physical therapy.[1,6,19,20]
  - Chiropractic treatment for chronic low back pain and chronic discogenic pain is controversial. The literature has few articles to support its use.[1,21]

- Sacroiliac and facet injections
  - Therapeutic low lumbar injections are common treatments for patients with back pain.
  - Although the literature is mixed and controversial, epidural steroid injections and selective nerve root blocks appear to be most effective for treating leg pain resulting from nerve root irritation; however, these treatments play a limited role in the treatment of low back pain.[1]
  - Facet injections, medial branch blocks, and rhizotomies have been used for the diagnosis and treatment of low back pain.[22-25] Unfortunately the literature is sparse, and some report that only 15% of patients with low back pain experience 50% or more relief, whereas 4% have complete relief.[24]
  - Sacroiliac joint injections can be used for the diagnosis and treatment of back pain emanating from the hip distal to the posterior iliac superior spine with normal, nonpainful range of motion of the hip.[23] Sacroiliac joint dysfunction commonly can be seen af-

ter lumbar fusion and presents in 15% to 30% of patients with chronic low back pain. Pain distal to the posterior superior iliac spine (PSIS), "radicular syndrome" without MRI or examination is evidence of root compression, and the combination of groin pain with buttock pain and a normal hip examination can be common findings.[23] Ninety percent sensitive and specific if "one-finger point test" to sacroiliac joint.

- During the FABER test, the hip and leg are flexed, abducted, and externally rotated; this position can isolate sacroiliac pathology. Back pain with this test is not considered diagnostic.
- Sacroiliac dysfunction is poorly correlated with history, radiographs, and physical examination findings, and should be diagnostically and therapeutically treated with injection.[22]
- Facet dysfunction or pain can be present in 3% of patients with failed back surgery[25] and in 15% to 40% of patients who have chronic low back pain.[22] The literature has noted variable correlation between history, physical examination, CT scans, and radiographs.[25]
- The diagnosis can be made with injections into the symptomatic joints. If this relieves the pain, then radiofrequency neurotomy may be considered.

Surgical

- Planning
  - See Pelvic Parameters, pp. 141 and 142.
  - See Intraoperative Management, Chapter 1, p. 2.
  - Bone Morphogenic Protein: An Evolving Role in Spine Surgery
    ‣ Bone morphogenic proteins (BMPs) are a group of transforming growth factors that belong to the transforming growth factor-beta (TGF-beta) superfamily. Originally discovered by Urist in 1965, extensive research has since evaluated the osteoinductive potential of this group of proteins. The osteoinductivity of BMPs supports the active recruitment

and proliferation of undifferentiated mesenchymal cells and the formation of osteoprogenitor cells with the capacity to form bone.[26] The osteoinductive potential of BMPs has made this an attractive alternative to iliac crest bone graft (ICBG) in spine fusion. Studies have shown complication rates of 10% to 50% with ICBG harvest.[27,28] ICBG harvest has been associated with morbidity, including ambulation difficulty, prolonged wound drainage and dehiscence, infection, unsightly scar, skin and buttock dysesthesia, prolonged operative times, increased cost, and pain.[27-29]

- In a consecutive series of 261 patients, Banwart, Asher, and Hassanein[28] reported a 10% major complication rate and a 39% minor complication rate after ICBG harvest.
- Sasso et al[27] reviewed prospective data on 208 patients with ICBG harvest for single-level anterior lumbar interbody fusion (ALIF). They found that 31% of patients had persistent pain 24 months after surgery, and 16% reported a fair to poor appearance of the graft harvest site.
- A cost analysis of 104 patients who underwent posterolateral lumbar spine fusion (52 with ICBG and 52 with recombinant human bone morphogenetic protein 2 [rhBMP-2]) found a total payer expenditure of $33,860 in the rhBMP-2 group and $37,227 in the ICBG group.[30]

▶ rhBMP-2 was approved for human use by the Food and Drug Administration as a bone graft substitute in 2002 after published studies showed its efficacy in ALIF.[31-33] rhBMP-2 was made commercially available as INFUSE (Medtronic, Memphis, TN). rhBMP-2 has been approved in a human dose of 1.5 mg/ml and for the specifics on label indication for use in a threaded intervertebral cage (LT-CAGE, Medtronic Sofamor Danek, Memphis, TN) on a type 1 bovine collagen sponge as a carrier during ALIF surgery.

- In a prospective, randomized, nonblinded study, 279 patients with symptomatic degenerative disc disease were randomly assigned to undergo ALIF with rhBMP-2 (143 patients) or ICBG (146 patients). Patients were followed for 24 months after surgery at these interval follow-up periods: 6 weeks and 3, 6, 12, and 24 months. Fusion was evaluated with plain radiographs and CT scans. There were similar improvements in outcomes in the Oswestry Disability Index (DOI), back pain, leg pain, and neurologic status at every interval follow-up point. At 24 months fusion rates were reported as 94.5% in the rhBMP-2 group and 88.7% in the ICBG group.[32,34]

▸ Because of the successful fusion rates and noted decrease in morbidity associated with ICBG harvest, the use of BMP as a bone graft substitute in spinal fusion increased rapidly. BMP usage increased from 0.7% of all fusion procedures in 2002 to 25% of all fusion procedures in 2006, with 85% used in single- or two-level fusions. In 2007 more than 50% of primary ALIFs, 43% of posterior lumbar interbody fusions/transforaminal lumbar interbody fusions (PLIFs/TLIFs), and 30% of PLFs were reported to use rhBMP-2.[35] This success has led to other studies evaluating the off-label use of BMP in posterolateral spinal fusion.

  - Prospective evaluation of 25 patients undergoing posterolateral spinal fusion randomly assigned to three treatment arms: ICBG/TSRH instrumentation (Medtronic Sofamor Danek) (5 patients), rhBMP-r/TSRH instrumentation (9 patients), and rhBMP-2 alone (11 patients). Patients were followed for an average of 17 months. The fusion rate was 40% (two of five) in the non-rhBMP-2 group and 100% in the groups with rhBMP-2. Improvement in the Oswestry score was seen at 6 weeks in the rhBMP-2–only group and at 3 months in the rhBMP-2/TSRH group. Improvement was not seen in the Oswestry group until 6 months in the autograft/TSRH group. At the final follow-up assessment, improvement in Oswestry score was greatest in the rhBMP-2-only group.[36]

- Meta-analysis of studies looking at the use of BMP in posterolateral fusion for degenerative disc disease of the lumbar spine: Seven studies and 331 patients were reviewed. The results revealed that BMPs were more effective than ICBG in achieving solid fusion, and rhBMP-2 was more effective than ICBG in promoting fusion, whereas rhBMP-7 (osteogenic protein-1) appeared equivalent to ICBG. Patients treated with BMPs had a shorter hospitalization compared with those who were treated with ICBG. BMPs appeared more efficient in instrumented fusions than in noninstrumented posterolateral fusions.[37]

- Dawson et al[38] performed a prospective, randomized, multicenter study comparing the use of rhBMP-2 on a collagen sponge along with an osteoconductive ceramic granule bulking agent and ICBG with instrumented posterolateral spinal fusion. At 24-month follow-up, the rhBMP-2 group showed a larger improvement in the ODI: 95% of patients in the rhBMP-2 group showed radiographic fusion compared with 70% in the ICBG group. The authors concluded that rhBMP-2 delivered on a type 1 collagen sponge may be an effective alternative to ICBG for single-level posterolateral fusion.

▸ Although there is evidence of the osteoinductive properties and the resultant benefits to spinal fusion, there are also associated complications. In a review published in 2002, Poynton and Lane[39] looked at the safety profile of BMP and its clinical use. They outlined a potential set of risks and recommendations, including the following:

- Bone overgrowth.
    - Inadvertent fusion at adjacent levels
    - Neural compression
    - Increased likelihood of bony overgrowth with exposed bone surfaces
    - Reconstitution of the lamina after laminectomy
    - Neural compression after foraminotomy
- No neural compression noted in posterolateral fusion in cases without laminectomy.
- No canal or foraminal stenosis after ALIF.[40]
- Increased risk of bony overgrowth in PLIF/TLIF procedures.
- The rhBMP-2 was better contained when delivered with a type 1 collagen sponge carrier.
- Recommendations:
    - The carrier (type 1 collagen sponge) and placement are important.
    - Avoid unnecessary exposure.
    - Apply bone wax to exposed bone surfaces.
    - Avoid irrigation of the wound after BMP placement.
▶ Other reported complications include[41-43]:
    - Epidural hematoma
    - Superficial and deep wound infections
    - Radiculitis
    - Ectopic bone formation
    - Retrograde ejaculation in male patients undergoing ALIF
    - Osteolysis
    - Graft subsidence and migration
    - Cyst formation
    - Urinary retention

- ◆ Catastrophic edema and airway compromise when used in the cervical spine
- ◆ A proposed increased risk of cancer
- ▶ Recent literature proposes that the original studies evaluating the efficacy of BMP and spinal fusion surgeries underreported the potential risks associated with the use of BMP as a substitute for ICBG.[44-46] In a 2011 study the literature associated with BMP was reviewed, and an increased risk of adverse events associated with rhBMP-2 was estimated at 10% to 50%. The results of this review are summarized as follows[46]:
  - ◆ PLIF/TLIF procedures: 25% to 50% risk of rhBMP-2 (1.5 mg/ml; INFUSE dose) associated adverse events, including osteolysis, graft migration, radiculitis, ectopic bone formation, and overall poorer global outcomes.
  - ◆ ALIF procedures: 10% to 15% risk of adverse events associated with rhBMP-2, including graft subsidence and displacement, infection, cyst formation, urinary retention, and retrograde ejaculation.
  - ◆ Anterior cervical procedures: 40% greater risk of adverse events in the acute postoperative period, including life-threatening complications.
  - ◆ Posterolateral fusion procedures: An equivalent or increased risk in the early postoperative period when compared with ICBG; 16% to 20% of patients had adverse back and leg pain and an increased risk of wound problems and cyst formation when rhBMP-2 was used.
- ▶ Two extensive systematic reviews recently published by independent evaluators looked at the safety and efficacy of rhBMP-2 in spinal fusion.[44] The initial study reviewed 11 of the original 17 studies on the industry-sponsored trials evaluating the role of rhBMP-2 in spinal fusion procedures. The results of this review revealed:

- ◆ ODI scores that were 3.5% lower in the rhBMP-2 group compared with ICBG.
- ◆ Fusion rate 12% higher in the rhBMP-2 group.
- ◆ Pain was more common shortly after surgery in the rhBMP-2 group.
- ◆ Cancer was more common after surgery with rhBMP-2, but the small number of patients with cancer made the cancer incidence inconclusive.

▶ The second study reviewed 13 randomized control trials and 31 cohort studies. The data were synthesized and the results reported.[45]

- ◆ In lumbar spine fusion, rhBMP-2 and ICBG were similar in overall success, fusion, and other effectiveness measures and in risk for any adverse events, although rates were high across interventions (77% to 93% at 24 months after surgery).
- ◆ In ALIF, rhBMP-2 was associated with an increased risk for retrograde ejaculation and urogenital problems, but this risk was not statistically significant.
- ◆ In anterior cervical spine fusion, rhBMP-2 was associated with increased risk for wound complications, swelling, airway compromise, and dysphagia.
- ◆ The cancer risk was increased with rhBMP-2, but cancer event rates were low and the types of cancer were heterogeneous.
- ◆ Overall the authors concluded that early journal publications did not correctly represent the efficacy and potential harm associated with rhBMP-2.
- ◆ In spinal fusion rhBMP-2 does not have a proven clinical advantage over ICBG and may be associated with potential risks.

▶ As noted in the studies cited previously, there has been concern about the risk of cancer with rhBMP-2. BMP receptors are present on different types of cancer and presumably could have an increased risk of tumorigenesis. In a retrospective cohort of Medicare beneficiaries who underwent lumbar fusion surgery, Cooper and Kou[47] found that 15.4% of patients treated with rhBMP-2 and 17% of those not treated with BMP developed a new cancer diagnosis, with an average follow-up of 4.7 years. The authors concluded that the use of rhBMP-2 is not associated with an increased risk of cancer.

- ▸ The overall role of BMP in spinal fusion continues to evolve. To date rhBMP-2 is FDA approved for use in the threaded LT-CAGE (Medtronic, Memphis, TN) in ALIF. The approved dose is 1.5 mg/ml (INFUSE, Medtronic). Other applications of rhBMP-2 in spine surgery may have a role in spinal fusion, but this use is considered off-label. When the use of rhBMP in spinal fusion procedures is planned, the potential risks should be discussed with the patient before surgery.
- Indications for surgery for degenerative disc disease
  - The North American Spine Society suggests the following indications:
    - ▸ Unremitting pain and disability for more than 6 months
    - ▸ Failure of a trial of aggressive conservative treatment lasting more than 4 months
    - ▸ MRI consistent with advanced disc degeneration
    - ▸ Concordant provocative discogram
    - ▸ Normal findings from a psychiatric evaluation
- Spondylolisthesis indications for surgery
  - Persistent back pain that interferes with activities of daily living and has failed conservative management.[48]
  - Significant progression of slip: The slip is >50% with a slip angle greater than 55 degrees.[48]
  - Neurologic deficit is present but does not respond to conservative management.

▪ Techniques
"Fusion is not the 'F' word"—*Scott Boden, MD*
- Fusion studies
  ▸ Between 1988 and 1990, more than 62,000 lumbar fusions were performed annually in the United States. The failure rate was reported to range from 20% to 40%.
  ▸ Turner et al[49] performed a metaanalysis of patient outcomes after lumbar fusion. Studies with more than 30 patients and a follow-up period longer than 1 year were included. The diagnoses included the following degenerative conditions: Disc herniation, internal disc derangement, degenerative scoliosis, segmental instability, pseudarthrosis, failed back surgery syndrome, spondylolisthesis, and spinal stenosis. The authors found, on average, a 68% satisfactory outcome after lumbar fusion. The results in terms of back pain relief were rated as good or excellent by 61% of the patients and poor or fair by 35%. Turner concluded that their analysis "did not support the superiority of any fusion procedure over others for clinical outcome." Their study supported the necessity of further prospective randomized controlled trials.
  ▸ Problems with Turner's metaanalysis[50]
    1. Reviewed articles published before much of the modern technology (i.e., pedicle fixation)
    2. Variety of diagnostic categories
    3. Review of the literature not a true meta-analysis
    4. Compared decompressive surgeries with decompressive surgeries with fusions
- Posterolateral fusion with graft alone
  ▸ Description/rationale
    ◆ Stabilize the motion segment with fusion and bone graft.
  ▸ Complications
    ◆ Pseudarthrosis ranges from 5% to 32%.[51,52]

- ▸ Results
  - ◆ 47% to 90% report good to fair results.[51,52]
- ▸ Concerns
  - ◆ Does not address the "pain generator" (the disc).[51,52]
  - ◆ Fusions in situ do not have the ability to correct alignment that instrumentation is able to correct.
  - ◆ The clinical success of fusion with graft alone lags behind fusion with instrumentation's success.
  - ◆ Iliac crest site morbidity versus the expense of bone graft substitutes and bone morphogenetic protein (BMP).[51,52]
- ▸ Studies
  - ◆ Weatherley et al[53] reported on five individuals who demonstrated on provocative discography reproduction of their symptoms in the discs treated with fusion. These patients experienced pain relief after undergoing anterior arthrodesis.
- • Posterolateral fusion with instrumentation
  - ▸ Description/rationale
    - ◆ Fusion with the addition of instrumentation improves the fusion rate. Zdeblick[54,55] found fusion rate improved by 30% when pedicle screws were added.
  - ▸ Complications
    - ◆ Related to screw placement
  - ▸ Results
    - ◆ Similar to that of noninstrumented fusion[51,52]
  - ▸ Concerns
    - ◆ Solid fusion does not always ensure a successful clinical outcome; adjacent-level disease might necessitate further fusions.[51,52]
    - ◆ Iliac crest site morbidity versus the expense of bone graft substitutes and BMP.
    - ◆ Fusion disease can result from a long incision, paraspinal muscle stripping, muscle ischemia during retraction, muscle

denervation if the transverse processes are exposed, persistent low back pain, extension weakness, and early lumbar fatigue.[54,55]

- ▶ Studies
  - ◆ Jackson et al[56] studied patients presenting with discogenic pain who had posterolateral fusion with instrumentation. They found an 87% fusion rate with 58% clinical success.
  - ◆ Zucherman et al[57] reported 89% fusion success and 60% clinical success.
- Posterior lumbar interbody fusion (PLIF)
  - ▶ Description/rationale
    - ◆ Provide global fusion through a posterior approach.
  - ▶ Results
    - ◆ Success ranges from 60% to 90%.[51,52]
  - ▶ Concerns
    - ◆ Destabilization of the motion segment.
    - ◆ During retraction of neural elements, a neural injury can occur.
    - ◆ Large amounts of scar and epidural fibrosis can make revision more difficult.[51,52]
    - ◆ Risk of dural tears, difficult to clear the disc space and restore lordosis, less structurally competent interbody device options (compared with ALIF), and destabilization of the anterior column (radical discectomy) and posterior column (radical decompression).[51,52]
  - ▶ Studies
    - ◆ Brantigan et al[58] studied 221 patients with different spinal pathologies who had PLIF augmented with posterior instrumentation. They reported a fusion rate of 96% and a clinical success rate of 86%. In the management of DDD in patients with a previous failed discectomy procedure, clinical success was achieved in 79 (86%) of 92 patients and arthrodesis in 91 (100%) of 91 patients.

- Anterior lumbar interbody fusion (ALIF)
  - ‣ Description/rationale
    - ◆ Removes the pain generator from an anterior approach only.

Red Flag: Anterior approach to the lumbar spine—before attempting anterior spine surgery, it is important to master the anterior approach technique.

- ‣ Anterior approach to lumbar spine
  A minimally invasive approach may be used for accessing the anterior lumbar spine. The iliac crest lateral and AP radiographs are used to plan the incision. For multiple levels, transitional level (may present with abnormal vascular anatomy), abnormal anatomy, and revisions, a vertical incision is used versus the horizontal, cosmetic incision. A retroperitoneal approach is used to approach the lumbar spine. The genitofemoral nerve and the sympathetic plexus consistently lie on the ventral surface of the psoas muscle, and if injured may result in testicular pain. At L5-S1 the left ureter is visible and should be retracted to the right. Once the iliac veins are visualized, blunt dissection is carried along the course of the medial edge of the left iliac vein, reflecting the prevertebral tissues toward the patient's right side. The dissection proceeds from left to right because the parasympathetic plexus is more adherent on the right side. Different levels of surgery have special considerations. For example, in the L5-S1 approach the superior hypogastric plexus may be injured and result in retrograde ejaculation. Only blunt dissection should be used and, if possible, monopolar electrocautery should be avoided. The middle sacral arteries are visible on the disc space and may have more than one artery present. Despite their appearing small in size, these arteries can present a problem if they

are not controlled, clipped, or tied. Initial retraction of the vessels will improve with disc removal, and more disc access can be obtained during the discectomy. Despite working in the bifurcation, the L5-S1 disc space is easier to approach versus the L4-5 space. During this approach, the vena cava may be tethered by the ascending iliolumbar vein, and this will need to be clipped or tied. This vein, at times, may be left if retraction can be safely done. Not controlling this vein can lead to serious bleeding problems if it is injured, and its vertical position makes gaining control difficult.

- ▶ Results
  - ◆ Zdeblick[55] reported a high fusion rate in 94% of patients with a Lumbar Threaded (LT) cage and in 100% of patients with an LT cage with rhBMP2 inside. He reported 85% to 90% clinical success. He found patient selection is critical to ensure success.
- ▶ Complications
  - ◆ Stand-alone cages suffered for the extraordinary use of cages during the "cage rage" era.[51,52]
  - ◆ Fusion is difficult to see.[52]
  - ◆ The construct might collapse and subside into endplates.[52]
  - ◆ Different success rates may occur when comparing L4-5 with L5-S1.
  - ◆ Tall discs might require posterior support.
  - ◆ Laparoscopic approach shows no advantage over mini-open approach.[59]
- • Transforaminal lumbar interbody fusion (TLIF)
  - ▶ Description/rationale
    - ◆ Provides posterior decompression and anterior-posterior stabilization without the risks of PLIF.[51,52] No approach surgeon is needed. Both columns are addressed through a single incision.

- ► Concerns
  - ◆ More difficult to obtain a complete disc excision compared with ALIF.
  - ◆ More difficult to reconstruct lordosis compared with ALIF.[51,52]
  - ◆ A calcified aorta prevents an anterior approach.
- ► Studies
  - ◆ Lowe et al[60] reported a 90% fusion rate and 79% good or excellent clinical outcome for patients treated by TLIF for a variety of lumbar pathologies (23 of 40 had DDD).
- • 360-degree fusion
  - ► Description/rationale
    - ◆ All pathology is fused and supported with anterior and posterior instrumentation.
  - ► Results
    - ◆ Slosar[61] studied 89 patients and reported a 99% fusion rate and 56% success rate in patients with DDD.
    - ◆ Moore et al[62] studied 58 patients and reported a 95% solid arthrodesis and 88% return to work; 86% of these patients had a "better" rating at 2-year follow-up.
  - ► Concerns
    - ◆ Because the fusion is both anterior and posterior, the 360-degree procedure can cause the breakdown of the adjacent segment. One should question the resorption of the posterior graft.[63]
    - ◆ Schwarzer et al[63] noted the posterior lateral lumbar fusion was solid on one side in 18% of patients studied and solid on both sides in 14% of patients studied. These poor PLF fusion rates in the presence of ALIF are consistent with the theory that when there is adequate anterior column support, the PLF may be deprived of the necessary biomechanical forces to fuse. This low rate of solid PLF is further support that a 270-degree fusion should function equivalently to the 360-degree fusion.[63]

- Far lateral surgery
  - ▸ Definition/rationale
    - ◆ A lateral retroperitoneal transpsoas approach with minimal muscle dissection through a tubular system and neuromonitoring
  - ▸ Anatomy
    - ◆ Lumbar plexus anatomy[64] (Fig. 9-1)
      - – Lateral femoral cutaneous nerve branches off the lumbar plexus at the level of the L3-4 foramen.
      - – Thirteen of 18 femoral nerves receive contributions from the L2-4 nerve roots and are formed at the L4-5 disc space.
      - – The femoral nerve is largest at the L4-5 disc space: 13 mm average.
    - ◆ Anatomy of compression
      - – AP diameter of L4 (34 mm).
      - – Retractor (three-prong) openings range from 20 to 30 mm.
      - – Femoral nerve 13 mm.

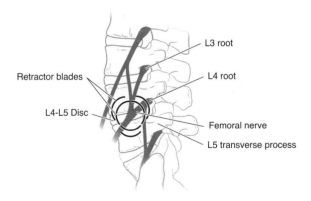

Fig. 9-1 Lateral retractor blades in relationship to transversing lumbar nerve roots.

- Opening the retractor to the posterior border of the disc space will result in compression from the retractor and transverse process.
- Compared with other transverse processes, the L5 transverse process is located ventrally.

♦ Nerves
- Park et al: The guidewire center of the L4-5 disc penetrated nerve tissue 15%, whereas 25% was within 8 mm of the nerve.
- Uribe et al reported that the genitofemoral nerve was at risk at the L2-3 disc space if the approach was anterior to the center of the disc.

Red Flag: Because nerve roots lack an epineurium and a perineurium, even small forces cause mechanical damage to nerve roots.

▸ Advantages
  ♦ Minimally invasive approach
    - Minimal muscle disruption
    - Shorter surgical time
    - Decreased blood loss
    - Decreased postoperative pain
    - Shorter admission time
    - Shorter recovery time
    - Similar or better long-term outcomes
  ♦ Benefits of a far lateral approach versus TLIF
    - Larger grafts.
    - No threat of bone growth into the canal using BMPs.
    - No ligamentous disruption: The far lateral approach uses intact anterior and posterior longitudinal ligaments for ligamentotaxic reduction.

  □ Through indirect decompression restoration of disc height and correction of alignment can be better achieved through ligamentotaxis created with the anterior and posterior longitudinal ligaments intact, because these exert great function on spinal alignment and stabilization.[65]

   ○ 41.9% increase in disc height

   ○ 13.5% increase in foraminal height

   ○ 24.7% increase in foraminal area

   ○ 33.1% increase in central canal diameter

  – No dural retraction with no irritation of the dorsal root ganglion causing radiculitis, scarring, and decompression.

  – Multilevel surgery through a smaller incision.

  – Less invasive with a smaller incision.

▶ Disadvantages

 ◆ Transpsoas: Postoperative thigh pain, weakness, and numbness

 ◆ Need for posterior fixation

 ◆ Neurapraxia at L4-5: Nerve irritation common at this level

 ◆ Long-term outcomes data lacking

 ◆ Fluoroscopy dependent

 ◆ Neuromonitoring a requirement

▶ Surgical indications

 ◆ Scoliosis: Using to attack the apex of the curve

 ◆ Flat-back syndrome: Sagittal imbalance

 ◆ Postlaminectomy syndrome with persistent stenosis

 ◆ Adjacent segment breakdown above a previous fusion

 ◆ Pseudarthrosis from a previous posterior instrumented fusion

 ◆ Foraminal stenosis

 ◆ Spondylolisthesis

 ◆ Symptomatic disc derangement in the thoracic and lumbar regions

- ▸ Contraindications to indirect decompression
  - ◆ Congenital stenosis or congenitally short pedicles
  - ◆ Uncontained disc herniation
  - ◆ Significant facet arthropathy with a calcified disc
  - ◆ Posterior longitudinal ligament or osteophytes arising from the posterior endplates with complete or near-complete compromise of the lateral recess
  - ◆ Synovial cysts
  - ◆ Radicular symptoms unimproved with flexion
- ▸ Preoperative planning
  - ◆ Check for unfavorable anatomy
    - – High iliac crest at L4-5
      - ▫ Consider AP and lateral radiographs.
      - ▫ More problematic in men.
    - – Long eleventh and twelfth ribs
      - ▫ Go intercostal or resect part of the ribs.
  - ◆ Approach considerations
    - – Left or right side is determined by choosing the side on which the patient has more leg symptoms.
    - – Choose the side that appears easiest to access on radiographs (e.g., resulting from crest, ribs, or scoliotic collapse).
    - – Correction can be equally good from either side; consider ease of access.
    - – Surgeon comfort.
- ▸ Technique
  - ◆ Patient positioning and positioning of the fluoroscopy equipment
    - – Position the patient with the side uppermost that has the most significant extremity pain.
    - – Place the patient's hips over the break in the table and place a hip roll underneath the hips.
    - – Place an axillary roll.

- Tape the patient's hip and chest down, running the tape perpendicular to the patient's body.
- Pushing the pelvis toward the foot of the table, run two diagonal tapes from the hip/pelvis to the corners of the bed; run another tape from the pelvis to the midportion of the foot of the bed, parallel to the bed. Add horizontal tape over the three tapes to the foot of the bed along the previously placed horizontal hip tape.
- Break the foot of the bed so that it pulls the pelvis and straightens the side of the torso that is uppermost.
- Bring in a fluoroscope; adjust the bed so the fluoroscope is parallel with or perpendicular to the floor. Adjust the patient as appropriate for fluoroscopic examination.
  - □ Perform an AP fluoroscopic view first.
    - ○ Adjust the bed by unlocking it, rotating to ensure that the endplates of the vertebral bodies are parallel.
    - ○ Adjust the tilt of the bed for rotation of the vertebral bodies.
  - □ Perform a lateral fluoroscopic view.
    - ○ Adjust the Trendelenburg position to ensure that the endplates are parallel.
- ◆ Mark the incision.
  - Work perpendicular to the floor.
  - Position the fluoroscope *before* draping the patient so true AP and lateral images will be obtained. If correction is needed, move the patient or table, *not* the fluoroscopy machine.
  - In multilevel cases readjust the *table* for perfect imaging at each level.
- ◆ Incision
  - Directly over the disc center for a single level
  - In between discs for two levels

- Dissection to the psoas muscle: Layers of the approach
  - Skin and subcutaneous tissue: Interabdominal nerves run through the muscles. If anatomic structures are injured with cautery, postoperative hernia or muscle atrophy can occur—a cosmesis issue.
  - Abdominal muscles: Use blunt dissection and minimal cautery when dissecting the external and internal oblique and transversalis abdominal muscles.
  - Retroperitoneal space: Follow the internal abdominal wall, and once posterior to the anterior abdominal wall, perform a finger sweep to feel for the quadratus muscle, transverse process, and surface of the psoas.
- Probe placement
  - Stimulate the probe to ensure the safety of the lumbar plexus.
  - Cover the tip with a finger and guide to the psoas to avoid puncturing the abdominal tissue.
  - Target the placement to the anterior one half to one third.
- Complications
  - Isaacs et al[66] reported the following complications:
    - One hundred seven patients underwent XLIF (eXtreme lateral interbody fusion) (NuVasive, San Diego, CA) for the treatment of degenerative scoliosis.
    - Mean operative time was 58 minutes per level, blood loss was 50 to 100 ml, 62.5% <100 ml.
    - 13 patients had major complications (12.1%) and 8 patients had minor complications.
  - Postoperative thigh symptoms
    - 1% to 60%
    - Transient versus 14% permanent[66]
    - Vague in defining thigh pain, weakness, and/or numbness
    - Trauma to psoas muscle versus femoral nerve stretch

- Youssef et al[67] reported the following complications in patients who underwent lateral approach interbody fusion:
  - Thirty-six patients (33.6%) had motor weakness, of which 86.2% resolved.
    - Statistically correlated with the length of surgery, not with the level treated or the number of levels.
    - Seven patients (6.5%) had weakness that did not resolve by 6 months or two motor grades.
    - All two-grade weakness resolved.
    - No statistical significance to any factor.
- Subsidence[68]
  - More challenging device placement results in an increase in the potential for subsidence.
  - Occurs in 14% of patients, but only 2.1% are clinically symptomatic.
    - Similar to PLIF, TLIF, and ALIF when BMP is used.
  - Higher when supplemental lateral plates are used, and lower when bilateral pedicle screws are used.
    - 70% occur at the superior endplate.
    - Inferior endplate is 40% stronger than the superior endplate.
    - Epiphyseal plates of the inferior endplates have a larger surface area than the superior endplates.
    - Endplate strength is weaker in the upper levels than in the lower levels.
  - Subsidence per level:
    - L1-2: 20%
    - L2-3: 10%
    - L3-4: 4%
    - L4-5: 10%
  - Subsidence and its relationship to the length of the construct:
    - 1: 10%

□ 2: 9%
□ 3: 25%
□ 4: 50%

> **Red Flag:** Over distraction plays a role in subsidence. Only 2 to 4 mm of distraction per level is required. Always downsize the implant.

- See Lumbopelvic fixation, pp. 146-148.
- Internal disc electrotherapy
  - ▸ Description/rationale
    - ◆ Coil is placed in disc to shrink collagen to reduce motion and destroy painful outer anulus fibers.
  - ▸ Concerns
    - ◆ Basic scientific studies do not support theory of benefit.[51]
    - ◆ Clinical results are mixed: Most studies do not show improvement over natural history; this technique is best performed on young, large discs, and results are only 50/50.[51]
  - ▸ Studies
    - ◆ Pro
      - – Saal and Saal[69] studied 25 patients; 80% reported a reduction of two points in the VAS for pain assessment and 72% discontinued pain medication.
      - – Karasek and Bogduk[70] found that 60% benefited after 1 year of treatment and 23% reported improvement in VAS scores compared with physical therapy control.
    - ◆ Con
      - – Freeman et al[71] performed a randomized, double-blind, controlled efficacy study of intradiscal electrotherapy (IDET) versus placebo. In the control group a probe was inserted into the disc, and the device was not activated for 16.5 minutes. The physician and patient were blind to group assignment. All patients completed a standardized

rehabilitation program; at 6-month follow-up, 55 of 57 patients had completed the study.
- Findings: No improvement on specific scales of SF-36, no improvement in Zung Depression Index (ZDI) or Modified Somatic Perceptions Questionnaire (MSPQ), and no significant improvement in either treatment group when comparing pretreatment with posttreatment scores. The authors concluded: "This study demonstrates no significant benefit from IDET over placebo."[71]

- Nucleus pulposus replacements
  - Description/rationale
    - Hydroactive implants mimic the nucleus pulposus by increasing their water content when the disc experiences decreased load.[72]
  - Complications
    - When implanted through a posterior approach, some implants extruded. This occurred less frequently when implantation was performed via an anterior approach.[72]
- Artificial disc
  - Description/rationale
    - Repair of the spinal column with the placement of implants that preserve/mimic the natural motion of the spine. Preservation of motion is considered to be superior for load distribution and damping effect. Motion preservation yields better functional results than arthrodesis.
  - Surgical indications for artificial disc replacement[73]
    - Prime candidates
      - 4 mm remaining disc height
      - No osteoarthritis changes to facet joints
      - No adjacent-level degeneration
      - Intact posterior elements

- Good candidates
  - 4 mm remaining disc height
  - No primary osteoarthritis changes to facet joints
  - Minimum degeneration of adjacent discs
  - Minimum posterior segment instability (e.g., postmicro-discectomy)
- Borderline candidates
  - <4 mm remaining disc height
  - Primary osteoarthritis changes to facet joints
  - Minimum adjacent-level degeneration
  - Minimum posterior segment instability
  - Adjacent to fusions
- Poor candidates
  - Gross degenerations of the spine
  - Secondary osteoarthritis changes to the facet joints
  - <4 mm disc height remaining at the adjacent levels
  - Posterior segment instability
- ▶ Results and prognosis for artificial disc replacement[74]
  - Lemaire studied 100 patients over 10 years after SB Charité device placement; good results remained in >80% of all cases. Poor results were attributed to incorrect indications in four cases—one with posterior facet arthritis, one with thoracolumbar kyphosis superior to the implant site, and two with extensive postoperative fibrosis.
  - Postoperative activity: Five patients retired and 82% returned to work; 72.7% have continued the same level activity (91.3% in the sedentary group; 66.6% in the light labor group; 83% in the heavy labor group).
  - Sixty-four patients had single- or multiple-level implantation of a total lumbar disc replacement between 1990 and 1993. The mean duration of follow-up was 8.7 years. At an average of 8.7 (range 7 to 11 years) years postoperatively, there were significant improvements in the back pain, radic-

ulopathy, disability, and modified Stauffer-Coventry scores; 80% of the patients had excellent or good results. Radiographs did not demonstrate loosening, migration, or mechanical failure in any patient. Five patients had approach-related complications.

▸ Concerns
  ◆ Two-year data still under investigation.
  ◆ "Disc rage" might occur, similar to the "cage rage" that occurred with anterior lumbar interbody cages when first introduced.
  ◆ A solid arthrodesis does not always result in a good clinical outcome.

DEGENERATIVE DISC DISEASE OUTCOMES
Diagnosis of Failed Back Surgery[75]

- Definitive diagnosis in 174 patients (94%)

Other Diagnoses

- Persistent foraminal stenosis 29%
- Painful discs 17%
- Pseudarthrosis 15%
- Recurrent disc herniation 6%
- Iatrogenic instability 5%
- Painful discs in fusion 3%
- These findings are also supported by Weatherley et al[76] and Barrick et al.[77]

Caraggee[78-82] Studies of 197 Patients

- Forty-six patients: Prospective, controlled study of the development of lower back pain in previously asymptomatic subjects undergoing experimental discography[78]
- Forty-two patients: Lumbar high-intensity zone and discography in subjects without low back pain[79]

- Thirty-two patients
  - A gold standard evaluation of the discogenic pain diagnosis as determined by provocative discography.[80]
  - The failure of surgery has a strong clinical effect in patients who had positive findings on discography and is rarely attributed to a primary misdiagnosis or poor patient selection.
  - This study had poor patient selection, which was noted when 6% of patients developed depression.
  - Poor surgical technique: 36% complication rate.
    - 10% reoperation to remove hardware
    - 6% narcotic withdrawal reaction
    - 6% vein laceration
    - 3% nonunion
- Eight patients
  - False-positive findings of lumbar discography[81]
- Sixty-nine patients
  - Low-pressure positive discography in subjects without symptoms of significant low back pain illness[82]

Swedish Lumbar Spine Study

- The Swedish Lumbar Spine Study Group[83] has done much to enrich the knowledge of the efficacy of lumbar fusion in the settling of discogenic back pain. In 2001 the group found that fusion for DDD results in superior outcomes compared with standard nonsurgical care. Moreover, using an incremental, cost-effectiveness ratio, the group showed that lumbar fusion, although initially more expensive, was a less expensive form of treatment in the long run than nonsurgical care. All of the treatment effects in that study were in favor of surgery.[84]

Literature Supports Fusion Surgery

- Although disc degeneration occurs frequently with aging and may be asymptomatic in most people, in certain instances it can cause severe low back pain. With reports of increases in spine surgery costs and volumes, pressures for cost containment have led to insurance company policies that limit coverage of fusion procedures. Although undisputedly there is room for more efficient provision of health care spending, the concern is growing that insurers' denials regarding spine fusion surgery are increasingly based on nontransparent guidelines provided by consulting firms without input from physicians, their respective societies, or evidence-based literature.

■ A Medline and Cochrane database search was performed to identify published articles reporting on validated patient-reported clinical outcome measures of 2 or more on the visual analog scale, ODI, short form health survey (SF-36), and patient satisfaction. A total of 26 articles were identified and stratified by the level of evidence; 18 of the 26 articles had level 1 data and a total of 3060 patients.

  • Studies of surgical versus nonsurgical treatment included six publications reporting on the results of prospective, randomized studies of fusion surgery versus nonsurgical therapy in patients with moderately severe pain. These studies included 547 patients who underwent fusions and 372 patients with nonsurgical therapy. The fusion groups had significant improvements in back pain, ODI, and satisfaction rates.

  • The weighted averages from the combined 3060 patients who underwent lumbar fusion across the 26 studies evaluated met or exceeded minimum clinically important differences on all patient-reported variables.

  • The body of literature supports fusion surgery as a viable treatment option for reducing pain and improving function in patients with chronic low back pain refractory to nonsurgical care when a diagnosis of disc degeneration can be made.[85] Improvement in pain and function was documented, with the degree of clinical improvement comparable with that seen in other common, well-accepted orthopedic procedures, such as total-knee replacement, hip revision, and spinal decompression surgery for spinal stenosis.[86]

- It is necessary to correctly identify patients with true discogenic pain, and it is imperative that all other sources of pain be excluded before performing surgery for discogenic back pain. In carefully selected patients, successful outcomes can be attained with surgical intervention.[87]

KEY POINTS

Before operating (fusion/artificial disc) for low back pain, review the classifications in Table 9-1 and consider the following.[51]

+ Don't operate on *black disc disease* without discography.[51]
+ Localize the pain source[51]; do not operate if unable to localize the pain.
+ Posterior rami of sinuvertebral nerve and other dorsal root branches innervate more than one vertebral segment.[51]
+ Imaging studies demonstrate abnormalities in asymptomatic subject.[51]
+ Provocative discography can be imprecise and results might be influenced by psychosocial issues/behavior.[17]
+ Most patients with degenerative low back pain improve without surgical treatment.[51]
+ A high percentage of patients with chronic axial pain have medicolegal or socioeconomic issues pending.[51]
+ Surgical results can be unpredictable.[51]
+ There is no consensus on the best method for treating chronic axial pain; however, numerous diagnostic and surgical techniques have been developed to provide options for treating patients with these debilitating conditions.[51]

✦ When one is performing far lateral surgery, it must be remembered that nerve roots lack an epineurium and a perineurium. Therefore even small forces cause mechanical damage to nerve roots.

✦ Over distraction plays a role in subsidence. Only 2 to 4 mm of distraction per level is required when performing far lateral surgery.

REFERENCES

1. Brodke D. Nonsurgical options for low back pain. Making the diagnosis. American Association of Orthopaedic Surgeons, Instructional Course, 2002.
2. Waddell G, McCulloch HA, Kummel E, et al. Non-organic physical signs in low-back pain. Spine 5:117-125, 1980.
3. Torstensen TA, Ljunggren AE, Meen HD, et al. Efficiency and costs of medical exercise therapy, conventional physiotherapy, and self-exercise in patients with chronic low back pain. A pragmatic, randomized, single-blinded, controlled trial with 1-year follow-up. Spine 23:2616-2624, 1998.
4. Flanagan MN, Chung BU. Roentgenographic changes in 188 patients 10-20 years after discography and chemonucleolysis. Spine 11:444-448, 1986.
5. Boden SD, McCowin PR, Davis DO, et al. Abnormal magnetic-resonance scans of the cervical spine in asymptomatic subjects. A prospective investigation. J Bone Joint Surg Am 72:1178-1184, 1990.
6. Andersen T, Chrisensen FB, Laursen M, et al. Smoking as a predictor of negative outcome in lumbar spinal fusion. Spine 26:2623-2628, 2001.
7. Anderson P. Low Back Pain. American Academy of Orthopaedic Surgeons Instructional Course, 2002. Rosemont, IL: The Academy, 2002.
8. Gaughen JR Jr, Jensen ME, Schweickert PA, et al. Relevance of antecedent venography in percutaneous vertebroplasty for the treatment of osteoporotic compression fractures. Am J Neuroradiol 23:594-600, 2002.
9. Derby R, Howard MW, Grant JM, et al. The ability of pressure-controlled discography to predict surgical and nonsurgical outcomes. Spine 24:364-371, 1999.
10. Johnson RG. Does discography injure normal discs? An analysis of repeat discograms. Spine 14:424-426, 1989.
11. Hinkley BS, Jaremko ME. Effects of 360-degree lumbar fusion in a workers' compensation population. Spine 22:312-322, 1997.
12. Colhoun E, McCall IW, Williams L, et al. Provocation discography as a guide to planning operations on the spine. J Bone Joint Surg Br 70:267-271, 1988.
13. Wiesel SW, Cuckler JM, DeLuca F, et al. Acute low back pain. An objective analysis of conservative therapy. Spine 5:324-330, 1980.

14. Deyo RA, Diehl AK, Rosenthal M. How many days of bed rest for acute low back pain? A randomized clinical trial. N Engl J Med 315:1064-1070, 1986.

15. Brooks P, Day RO. Non-steroidal antiinflammatory drugs—differences and similarities. N Engl J Med 324:1716-1725, 1991.

16. Cooper SA, Precheur H, Rauch D, et al. Evaluation of oxycodone and acetaminophen in treatment of postoperative dental pain. Oral Surg Oral Med Oral Pathol 50:496-501, 1980.

17. Donelson R, Grant W, Kamps C, et al. Pain response to sagittal end-range spinal motion. A prospective, randomized, multicentered trial. Spine 16:635-637, 1991.

18. Stankovic R, Johnell O. Conservative treatment of acute low-back pain. A prospective randomized trial: McKenzie method of treatment versus patient education in "mini back school." Spine 15:120-123, 1990.

19. Koes BW, Bouter LM, van Mameren H, et al. The effectiveness of manual therapy, physiotherapy, and treatment by the general practitioner for non-specific back and neck complaints. A randomized clinical trial. Spine 17:28-35, 1992.

20. Shekelle PG. Spine update: Spinal manipulation. Spine 19:858-861, 1994.

21. Bolender NF, Schonstrom NS, Spengler DM. Role of computed tomography and myelography in the diagnosis of central spinal stenosis. J Bone Joint Surg Am 67:240-246, 1985.

22. Dreyfuss P, Michaelsen M, Pauza K, et al. The value of medical history and physical examination in diagnosing sacroiliac joint pain. Spine 21:594-602, 1996.

23. Schofferman J. A prospective randomized comparison of 270 degree fusions to 360 degree fusions (circumferential fusions). Spine 26:E207-E212, 2001.

24. Schwarzer AC, Aprill CN, Bogduk N. The sacroiliac joint in chronic low back pain. Spine 20:31-37, 1995.

25. Schwarzer AC, Aprill CN, Derby R, et al. Clinical features of patients with pain stemming from the lumbar zygapophyseal joints. Is the lumbar facet syndrome a clinical entity? Spine 19:1132-1137, 1994.

26. Carlisle E, Fischgrund JS. Bone morphogenetic proteins for spinal fusion. Spine J 5(Suppl):S240-S249, 2005.

27. Sasso RC, LeHuec JC, Shaffrey C; and the Spine Interbody Group. Iliac crest bone graft donor site pain after anterior lumbar interbody fusion: A prospective patient satisfaction outcome assessment. J Spinal Disord Tech 18(Suppl):S77-S81, 2005.

28. Banwart JC, Asher MA, Hassanein RS. Iliac crest bone graft harvest donor site morbidity: A statistical evaluation. Spine 20:1055-1060, 1995.

29. Dimar JR, Glassman SD, Burkus KJ, et al. Clinical outcomes and fusion success at 2 years of single-level instrumented posterolateral fusions with recombinant human bone morphogenetic protein-2/compression resistant matrix versus iliac crest bone graft. Spine 31:2534-2540, 2006.

30. Carreon LY, Glassman SD, Djurasovic M, et al. RhBMP-2 versus iliac crest bone graft for lumbar spine fusion in patients over 60 years of age: A cost-utility study. Spine 34:238-243, 2009.

31. Boden SD, Zdeblick TA, Sandhu HS, et al. The use of rhBMP-2 in interbody fusion cages. Definitive evidence of osteoinduction in humans: a preliminary report. Spine 25:376-381, 2000.

32. Burkus JK, Gornet MF, Dickman CA, et al. Anterior lumbar interbody fusion using rhBMP-2 with tapered interbody cages. J Spinal Disord Tech 15:337-349, 2002.

33. Glassman SD, Carreon LY, Djurasovic M, et al. RhBMP-2 versus iliac crest bone graft for lumbar spine fusion. Spine 33:2843-2849, 2008.

34. Smoljanovic T, Siric F, Bojanic I. Six-year outcomes of anterior lumbar interbody arthrodesis with use of interbody fusion cages and recombinant human bone morphogenetic protein-2. J Bone Joint Surg Am 92:2614-2615, 2010.

35. Ong KL, Villarraga ML, Lau E, et al. Off-label use of bone morphogenetic proteins in the United States using administrative data. Spine 35:1794-1800, 2010.

36. Boden SD, Kang J, Sandhu H, et al. Use of recombinant human bone morphogenetic protein-2 to achieve posterolateral lumbar spine fusion in humans: A prospective, randomized clinical pilot trial: 2002 Volvo Award in Clinical Studies. Spine 27:2662-2673, 2002.

37. Papakostidis C, Kontakis G, Bhandari M, et al. Efficacy of autologous iliac crest bone graft and bone morphogenetic proteins for posterolateral fusion of lumbar spine: A meta-analysis of the results. Spine 33:E680-E692, 2008.

38. Dawson E, Bae HW, Burkus JK, et al. Recombinant human bone morphogenetic protein-2 on an absorbable collagen sponge with an osteoconductive bulking agent in posterolateral arthrodesis with instrumentation: A prospective randomized trial. J Bone Joint Surg Am 91:1604-1613, 2009.

39. Poynton AR, Lane JM. Safety profile for the clinical use of bone morphogenetic proteins in the spine. Spine 27(16 Suppl 1):S40-S48, 2002.

40. Deyo RA, Ching A, Matsen L, et al. Use of bone morphogenetic proteins in spinal fusion surgery for older adults with lumbar stenosis: Trends, complications, repeat surgery, and charges. Spine 37:222-230, 2012.

41. Williams BJ, Smith JS, Fu K-M, et al. Complications associated with BMP use in 11933 cases of spinal fusion. Spine J 10(Suppl 1):S98-S99, 2010.

42. Vaidya R, Sethi A, Bartol S, et al. Complications in the use of rhBMP-2 in PEEK cages for interbody spinal fusions. J Spinal Disord Tech 21:557-562, 2008.

43. Pradhan BB, Bae HW, Dawson EG, et al. Graft resorption with the use of bone morphogenetic protein: Lessons from anterior lumbar interbody fusion using femoral ring allografts and recombinant human bone morphogenetic protein-2. Spine 31:E277-E284, 2006.

44. Simmonds MC, Brown J, Heirs MK, et al. Safety and effectiveness of recombinant human bone morphogenetic protein-2 for spinal fusion: A meta-analysis of individual-participant data. Ann Intern Med 158:877-889, 2013.

45. Fu R, Selph S, McDonagh M, et al. Effectiveness and harms of recombinant human bone morphogenetic protein-2 in spine fusion: A systemic review and meta-analysis. Ann Intern Med 158:890-902, 2013.

46. Carragee EJ, Hurwitz EL, Weiner BK. A critical review of recombinant human bone morphogenetic protein-2 trials in spinal surgery: Emerging safety concerns and lessons learned. Spine J 11:471-491, 2011.

47. Cooper GS, Kou TD. Risk of cancer after lumbar fusion surgery with recombinant human bone morphogenetic protein-2. Spine 38:1862-1868, 2013.

48. Miller MD. Review of Orthopaedics, 3rd ed. Philadelphia: WB Saunders, 2000.

49. Turner JA, Ersek M, Herron L, et al. Patient outcomes after lumbar spinal fusions. JAMA 268:907-911, 1992.

50. Hilibrand AS, Rand N. Degenerative lumbar stenosis: Diagnosis and treatment. J Am Acad Orthop Surg 7:239-249, 1999.

51. Glassman SD, Rose SM, Dimar JR, et al. The effect of postoperative nonsteroidal anti-inflammatory drug administration on spinal fusion. Spine 23: 834-838, 1998.

52. Herkowitz H. Surgical Options for "Discogenic" Low Back Pain. American Academy of Orthopaedic Surgery Instructional Course, 2002. Rosemont, IL: The Academy, 2002.

53. Weatherley CR, Prickett CF, O'Brien JP. Discogenic pain persisting despite solid posterior fusion. J Bone Joint Surg Br 68:142-143, 1986.

54. Zdeblick T. The surgical treatment of back pain. Presented at the Annual Meeting of the American Academy of Orthopaedic Surgeons, New Orleans, Feb 2003.

55. Zdeblick TA. A prospective, randomized study of lumbar fusion: Preliminary results. Spine 18:983-991, 1993.

56. Jackson RK, Boston DA, Edge AJ. Lateral mass fusion. A prospective study of a consecutive series with long-term follow-up. Spine 10:828-832, 1985.

57. Zucherman J, Hsu K, Picetti G III, et al. Clinical efficacy of spinal instrumentation in lumbar degenerative disc disease. Spine 17:834-837, 1992.

58. Brantigan JW, Steffee AD, Lewis ML, et al. Lumbar interbody fusion using the Brantigan I/F cage for posterior lumbar interbody fusion and the variable pedicle screw placement system: Two-year results from a Food and Drug Administration investigational device exemption clinical trial. Spine 25:1437-1446, 2000.

59. Zdeblick TA, David SM. A prospective comparison of surgical approach for anterior L4-L5 fusion. Spine 25:2682-2687, 2000.

60. Lowe TG, Tahernia AD, O'Brien MF, et al. Unilateral transforaminal posterior lumbar interbody fusion (TLIF): Indications, technique, and 2-year results. J Spinal Disord Tech 15:31-38, 2002.

61. Slosar PJ. Indications and outcomes of reconstructive surgery in chronic pain of spinal origin. Spine 27:2555-2562, 2002.

62. Moore KR, Pinto MR, Butler LM. Degenerative disc disease treated with combined anterior and posterior arthrodesis and posterior instrumentation. Spine 27:1680-1686, 2002.

63. Schwarzer AC, Aprill CN, Derby R, et al. The false-positive rate of uncontrolled diagnostic blocks of the lumbar zygapophyseal joints. Pain 58:195-200, 1994.

64. Davis TT, Bae HW, Mok JM. Lumbar plexus anatomy within the psoas muscle: Implications for the transpsoas lateral approach to the L4-L5 disc. J Bone Joint Surg Am 93:1482-1487, 2011.

65. Oliveira L, Marchi L, Coutinho E, et al. A radiographic assessment of the ability of the extreme lateral interbody fusion procedure to indirectly decompress neural elements. Spine 35(26 Suppl):S331-S337, 2010.

66. Isaacs RE, Hyde J, Goodrich A, et al. A prospective, nonrandomized, multicenter evaluation of extreme lateral interbody fusion for the treatment of adult degenerative scoliosis: Perioperative outcomes and complications. Spine 35(26 Suppl):S322-S330, 2010.

67. Youssef JA, McAfee PC, Patty CA, et al. Minimally invasive surgery: Lateral approach interbody fusion: Results and review. Spine 35(26 Suppl):S302-S311, 2010.

68. Le TV, Baaj AA, Dakwar E, et al. Subsidence of polyether ether ketone intervertebral cages in minimally invasive lateral retroperitoneal transpsoas lumbar interbody fusion. Spine 37:1268-1273, 2012.

69. Saal JS, Saal JA. Management of chronic discogenic low back pain with a thermal intradiscal catheter. A preliminary report. Spine 25:382-388, 2000.

70. Karasek M, Bogduk N. Twelve-month follow-up of a controlled trial of intradiscal thermal anuloplasty for back pain due to internal disc disruption. Spine 25:2601-2607, 2000.

71. Freeman BJC, Fraser RD, Christopher MJ, et al. A randomized, double-blind, controlled trial: Intradiscal electrothermal therapy versus placebo for the treatment of chronic discogenic low back pain. Spine 30:2369-2377, 2005.

72. Eysel P, Rompe J, Schoenmayr R, et al. Biomechanical behavior of a prosthetic lumbar nucleus. Acta Neurochir 141:1083-1087, 1999.

73. Bertagnoli R, Kumar S. Indications for full prosthetic disc arthroplasty: A correlation of clinical outcome against a variety of indications. Eur Spine J 11(Suppl 2):S131-S136, 2002.

74. Tropiano P, Huang RC, Girardi FP, et al. Lumbar total disc replacement. Seven to eleven-year follow-up. J Bone Joint Surg Am 87:490-496, 2005.

75. Waquespack A, Schofferman J, Slosar P, et al. Etiology of long-term failures of lumbar spine surgery. Pain Med 3:18-22, 2002.
76. Weatherley CR, Prickett CF, O'Brien JP. Discogenic pain persisting despite solid posterior fusion. J Bone Joint Surg Br 68:142-143, 1986.
77. Barrick WT, Schofferman JA, Reynolds JB, et al. Anterior lumbar fusion improves discogenic pain at levels of prior posterolateral fusion. Spine 25:853-857, 2000.
78. Carragee EJ, Barcohana B, Alamin T, et al. Prospective controlled study of the development of lower back pain in previously asymptomatic subjects undergoing experimental discography. Spine 29:1112-1117, 2004.
79. Carragee EJ, Paragioudakis SJ, Khurana S. 2000 Volvo Award winner in clinical studies: Lumbar high-intensity zone and discography in subjects without low back problems. Spine 25:2987-2992, 2000.
80. Carragee EJ, Lincoln T, Parmar VS, et al. A gold standard evaluation of the "discogenic pain" diagnosis as determined by provocative discography. Spine 31:2115-2123, 2006.
81. Carragee EJ, Tanner CM, Yang B, et al. False-positive findings on lumbar discography. Reliability of subjective concordance assessment during provocative disc injection. Spine 24: 2542-2547, 1999.
82. Carraggee EJ, Alamin TF, Carragee JM. Low-pressure positive discography in subjects asymptomatic of significant low back pain illness. Spine 31:505-509, 2006.
83. Fritzell P, Hagg O, Wessberg P, et al.; Swedish Lumbar Spine Study Group. 2001 Volvo Award Winner in Clinical Studies: Lumbar fusion versus nonsurgical treatment for chronic low back pain: A multicenter prospective randomized controlled trial from the Swedish Lumbar Spine Study Group. Spine 26:2521-2532, 2001.
84. Fritzell P, Hagg O, Jonsson D, et al.; Swedish Lumbar Spine Study Group. Cost-effectiveness of lumbar fusion and nonsurgical treatment for chronic low back pain in the Swedish Lumbar Spine Study: A multicenter, randomized, controlled trial from the Swedish Lumbar Spine Study Group. Spine 29:421-434, 2004.
85. Phillips FM, Slosar PJ, Youssef JA, et al. Lumbar spine fusion for chronic low back pain due to degenerative disc disease: A systematic review. Spine 38: E409-E422, 2013.
86. Hansson T, Hansson E, Malchau H. Utility of spine surgery: A comparison of common elective orthopaedic surgical procedures. Spine 33:2819-2830, 2008.
87. Madigan L, Vaccaro AR, Spector LR. Management of symptomatic lumbar degenerative disk disease. J Am Acad Orthop Surg 17:102-111, 2009.

10 ▪ Spinal Stenosis

Stenosis is the narrowing of the space through which neural elements run. As abnormal motion develops within a degenerated motion segment, it exacerbates nerve root irritation in the stenotic lateral recess and foramen.[1] Types of spinal stenosis include the following:

- Central spinal stenosis
  - Commonly occurs at the disc level as a result of overgrowth in the facet joint region (mainly involving the inferior articular process of the cephalad vertebra) and thickening and redundancy of the ligamentum flavum (Fig. 10-1).[1]
- Lateral recess
- Foraminal
- Congenital
- Spondylolytic
- Hardware compression

Red Flag: A trefoil-shaped canal increases the risk of lateral recess stenosis.[2]

SIGNS AND SYMPTOMS

- Patients are usually 50 to 60 years old and complain of gradual onset of low back pain[2]
- Patients may present with radicular-type symptoms or neurogenic pain. Neurogenic pain can present as pain to the coccyx, buttocks, and posterior thighs with cramping and tightness with activities.[1]

- Symptoms may be relieved with flexion. Symptoms are usually exacerbated by standing, walking, and exercising in an erect posture, which results in the development of pain, tightness, heaviness, and subjective weakness in the legs.[1,2] This symptom complex is referred to as *neurogenic claudication* and is rapidly relieved by sitting down or leaning forward (Table 10-1).[1,2]

Fig. 10-1   Anatomic grid pattern for evaluating lumbar spinal stenosis. **A,** Posterior cutaway view shows the relationship of the neural elements to the five sagittal zones and the three repeating transverse levels. **B,** Posterior view with the posterior elements intact shows the relationship of the facet joints and the pars interarticularis to the neural elements and the anatomic grid pattern. (Modified from Spivak JM. Degenerative lumbar spinal stenosis [review]. J Bone Joint Surg Am 80:1053-1066, 1998.)

Table 10-1 Symptom Comparison of Neurogenic and Vascular Claudication

	Vascular	Neurogenic
Claudication distance	Fixed	Variable
Relief after stop walking	Immediate	Slow
Relief of pain	Standing	Sitting
Walk uphill	Pain	No pain
Bicycle ride	Pain	No pain
Type of pain	Cramping	Numbness, ache
Radiation	Distal → proximal	Proximal → distal
Pulses	Absent, diminished	Present

CLINICAL EVALUATION
Physical Examination

- Patients may have a fairly benign presentation.
- Patients may have a stooped-forward gait and rarely will have motor deficits.
- A sac narrower than 10 mm is usually associated with clinical symptoms.[1]
- Amundsen et al[3] demonstrated that the most common symptoms of lumbar stenosis include back pain (95%), claudication (91%), leg pain (71%), weakness (33%), and voiding disturbances (12%). The radicular pattern or pain pattern corresponded to the L5 root in 91% of patients, S1 in 63%, L1-4 in 28%, and S2-5 in 5%. Forty-seven percent of patients had double root involvement, 17% had triple root involvement, and 35% had single root involvement. Fifty-one percent had sensory changes, 47% had reflex changes, 40% had lumbar tenderness, 36% had reduced spinal mobility, 24% had a positive straight leg raise, and 6% had perianal numbness.

WORKUP

> **Red Flag:** As we age, degenerative changes are common in the lumbar spine. Patients may be asymptomatic.

Radiographs

- Degenerative changes are common. The source of the pain may be difficult to diagnose.
- Flexion-extension radiographs: Look for instability.
- Anteroposterior radiographs: Look for scoliosis.

CT/Myelogram

- Best study for visualizing neural compression.
- Postmyelographic CT is superior to MRI as a single study for pre-operative planning of decompression of lumbar spinal stenosis.[2]
  - Trefoil-shaped canals have the smallest cross-sectional area and are associated with the highest incidence of symptomatic lumbar stenosis.[4]
  - Nerve root entrapment in the lateral recess or central canal stenosis is demonstrated by the level of cutoff of contrast material.[1]
  - A sac narrower than 10 mm was usually associated with clinical symptoms.[1]

Electromyography/Nerve Conduction Velocity

- Used to differentiate spinal stenosis from peripheral neuropathy, which is caused by diabetes and affects the peripheral motor and sensory nerves.
- Test may be subjective because the results depend on the experience of the technician.[5]
- Polyradiculopathy, often with bilateral involvement of multiple levels, is a typical pattern in symptomatic patients.

- Evaluation of somatosensory evoked potentials before and after exercise may help determine which nerve roots are most involved in central spinal canal stenosis at the lumbar level.[5]

TREATMENT/MANAGEMENT
Nonsurgical (Fig. 10-2)

- Bracing
  - Found to be effective for treatment of painful spondylolisthesis.
- Limited activity, physical therapy, NSAIDs, epidural steroids
  - Bicycle riding has been found to be a good activity.
  - Epidural steroid injections (see Lumbar Radiculopathy, Chapter 7, pp. 155 and 156).
    - ▸ Efficacy of epidural steroid injections, on average, <3 months[6]
    - ▸ Epidural steroid injections not as precise as transforaminal epidural steroid injections in delivering medication to target tissues[6]

    If the first injection provides symptomatic relief, one or two additional injections are prescribed. If *no* benefit is experienced after one injection, injection treatment should be discontinued.
  - The literature contains conflicting reports concerning the value of injections.
    - ▸ Cuckler et al,[7] in a prospective, randomized, double-blind study, found no statistically significant difference in symptomatic improvement with placebo injections.
    - ▸ Dilke et al[8] demonstrated a significant improvement in short-term pain and functional measurements.
    - ▸ Holt[9] noted that 48% of patients demonstrated functional improvement 2 years after injection.
    - ▸ Vertebral osteophytes that bridge spinal segments and narrow disc spaces may signify that there has been some spontaneous stability provided in the region of the degenerative spinal stenosis and asymmetrical collapse.[5] As a general rule, the greater the disc height, the greater the motion that the segment has

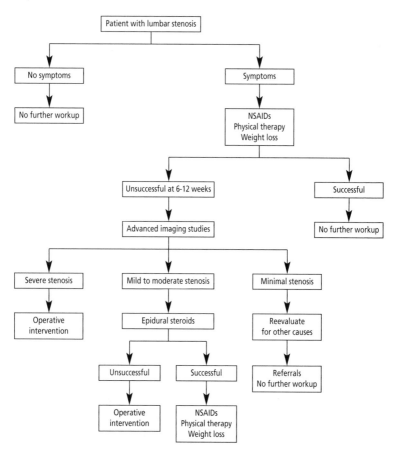

Fig. 10-2 Algorithm for nonoperative management of degenerative lumbar stenosis. (From Hilibrand AS. Degenerative lumbar stenosis. Diagnosis and treatment. J Am Acad Orthop Surg 7:239-249, 1999.)

remaining, meaning a collapsed disc with osteophytes is at relatively low risk for progression, and one might be able to perform a laminectomy alone or a fusion without instrumentation. In some instances, a single symptomatic nerve root can be isolated by means of selective diagnostic injections, allowing for a more limited decompression. This also may obviate the need for arthrodesis, especially in a patient who has had no back pain or history of marked progression of the deformity.[5]

Surgical (Fig. 10-3)

- Indications
  - Failure of nonsurgical treatment
  - Predominantly back/leg pain
  - Restriction of activities of daily living
  - Confirming imaging studies

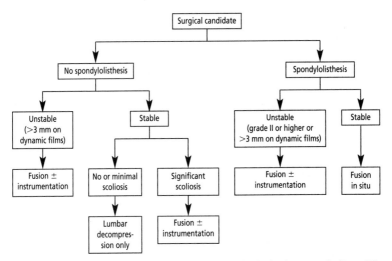

Fig. 10-3 Algorithm for surgical management of degenerative lumbar stenosis. (From Hilibrand AS. Degenerative lumbar stenosis. Diagnosis and treatment. J Am Acad Orthop Surg 7:239-249, 1999.)

- Techniques
  - Techniques vary from minimal decompression without fusion to wide decompression with instrumented fusion.
- Technical considerations
  - Decompressive lumbar laminectomy is most stenotic at the facet level. The hypertrophic ligamentum flavum must be removed.[1]
  - During lateral recess decompression (partial medial facetectomy), preserve at least 50% of the facet joint surface area and approximately 1 cm of the dorsal surface of the pars.
  - Reasons for arthrodesis included instability (transitional or iatrogenic), spondylolysis, and scoliosis.[1]
- Additional considerations for lumbar stenosis
  - Stenosis with degenerative spondylolisthesis
    ‣ The anterior vertebral subluxation results in severe narrowing of the spinal canal between the inferior aspect of the lamina and inferior articular process of the fourth lumbar vertebra and the superior aspect of the posterior portion of the fifth lumbar vertebral body.[5]
    ‣ Usually seen at L4-5, sagittal facets may increase the risk of slippage and may only be seen on flexion-extension radiographs.
  - Stenosis with scoliosis
    ‣ Adult degenerative scoliosis develops as a result of asymmetrical narrowing of the disc space and vertebral rotation secondary to the instability caused by disc degeneration.[5,10,11]
    ‣ Collapse in the concavity results in narrowing of the neural foramen between adjacent pedicles. As a result, symptoms on the anterior thigh and leg (resulting from compression of the cephalad and middle lumbar nerve roots) are more common on the side of the concavity of the major lumbar curve.[7]
    ‣ Radiating pain in the posterior portion of the lower extremity is more common on the side of the convexity of the lumbar

curve; such pain is due to compression of the caudad lumbar nerve roots and the sacral nerve roots.[1,5]

▸ Indications for fusion to treat scoliosis: Curve >35 degrees, lateral listhesis, and documented curve progression (Fig. 10-4).[10,11]

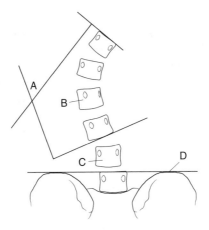

Fig. 10-4   Risk factors for lumbar curve progression. *A,* Cobb angle ≥30 degrees; *B,* apical rotation ≥ grade II (Nash-Moe); *C,* lateral listhesis ≥6 mm; *D,* intercrest line through or below L4-5 disc space. (Modified from Tribus CB. Degenerative lumbar scoliosis. Evaluation and management [review]. J Am Acad Orthop Surg 11:174-183, 2003.)

- Stenosis with lumbar kyphosis
    - ▸ The sagittal plane should always be considered.
    - ▸ In patients with preoperative sagittal imbalance from loss of lordosis as a result of disc space collapse, consideration should be given to anterior or posterior lumbar discectomies with structural interbody bone-grafting to restore disc height and lordosis should be considered before posterior decompression and stabilization.[5]

- Recurrent spinal stenosis
  - ▸ Bone regrowth with recurrent stenosis may be seen more frequently in association with decompression involving limited resection of bone.[5]
- Intraoperative structural alteration
  - ▸ Excessive facet removal: Preserve at least 50% of the two facets.[1]
  - ▸ Pars excision: Leave at least 1 cm of the pars.[1]
- Stenosis with postlaminectomy instability (Fig. 10-5)
  - ▸ When radiographic findings reveal postlaminectomy instability, procedures that do not include some type of fusion will fail to solve the problem; wider decompression or discectomy alone will only further destabilize the segment.[10-12]

Fig. 10-5 Criteria of instability. In functional lateral radiographs: Rotatory hypermobility >15 degrees, >3 mm anterior translation, and >3 mm posterior translation. In static anteroposterior radiographs: Disc wedging >5 degrees and >3 mm lateral translation. (From Aota Y, Kumana K, Hirabuyashi S. Post fusion instability of the adjacent segments after rigid pedicle screw fixation for degenerative lumbar spine disorders. J Spinal Disorders 18:464-473, 1995.)

POSSIBLE PREDICTORS OF POOR OUTCOMES
Back Pain as Predominant Symptom

- These patients are less likely to be satisfied after operative decompression than those patients who present with symptoms predominantly in the lower extremities, even if spinal stenosis is found on an advanced imaging study.[5] Back pain often results from muscle fatigue secondary to the forward flexed position.

Transitional Syndrome

- Progression of spondylolisthesis can occur even when concomitant arthrodesis without instrumentation is performed.[10,11] Preoperative radiographic and anatomic risk factors associated with the postoperative development or progression of spondylolisthesis at L4-5 include a well-maintained disc height, absence of degenerative osteophytes, and a smaller, sagittally oriented facet joint.[5]

Comorbid Conditions

- Diabetes, osteoarthritis of hip, preoperative fracture of a lumbar vertebra, and preoperative degenerative scoliosis[5]

Infection (Fig. 10-6)

- Low incidence of infection if the proper surgical technique is used as well as preoperative antibiotics and irrigation during the procedure

Smoking

- Several studies have shown the negative effects of nicotine on the success of lumbar spinal fusion.
  - Andersen et al[13,14] noted that the reason for the negative effects could be that nicotine hinders the early revascularization of bone graft, probably exerted by downregulated gene transcription of

Fig. 10-6 Algorithm for surgical treatment of spinal infections. (From Hadjipavlou AG. Algorithm for surgical intervention of pyogenic spinal infection. Spine 25:1668-1679, 2000.)

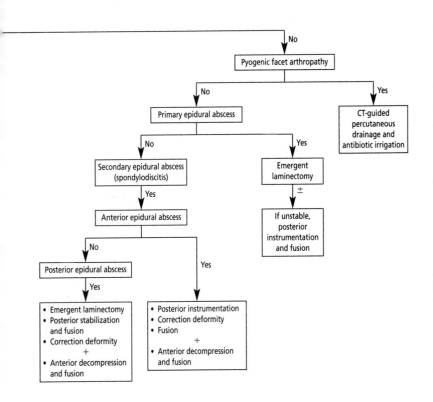

fibroblast growth factor basic, vascular endothelial growth factor, and BMP: Cytokines known to be important in relation to angiogenesis and osteoblast function.[13,14] This is supported by experimental models that noted cessation of the nicotine exposure before surgery improved fusion rates.

- Interestingly, in reviews of spondylolisthesis fusions[15] and scoliosis fusions,[16] no significant benefit from preoperative smoking cessation was shown. However, postoperative smoking correlated with a significantly increased rate of pseudarthrosis.[12,15] Cessation of smoking with the use of nicotine substitutes is not beneficial because animal studies and human clinical trials have shown that nicotine is a major factor in failure of fusion in patients who continue to smoke.[14]

- Andersen et al[13] found preoperative smoking to be a significant predictor of fusion failure (double the pseudarthrosis rate) in lumbar spinal fusion surgery. Postoperative smoking cessation for 6 months after the fusion procedure increased the fusion rate to a level comparable with that of nonsmokers.[13,14]

- Furthermore, Snider et al[17] found that smoking was negatively related to fusion, but a stronger correlation was found between fusion and general physical and socioeconomic factors.

NSAIDs and Pseudarthrosis (Fig. 10-7)

- Decreasing narcotic use for postoperative pain management has experienced a rise in popularity.

- Glassman et al[16] reported 29 cases of pseudarthrosis in 167 patients when ketorolac was used as a postoperative analgesic, whereas only five fusion failures were noted in 121 patients not using ketorolac. Indomethacin and ibuprofen have been shown to adversely affect bone formation in clinical and animal trials.[14]

- Martin et al[18] performed an animal study that confirmed the detrimental effects of spinal fusion during the immediate postoperative period after posterolateral lumbar spinal fusion. They reported

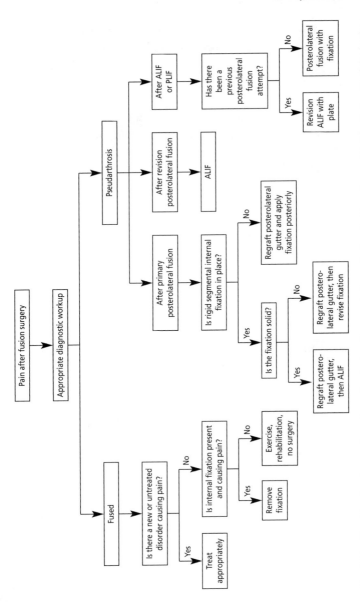

Fig. 10-7 Algorithm for diagnostic workup of patients with suspected pseudarthrosis. (From Larsen JM. Pseudarthrosis of the lumbar spine. J Am Acad Orthop Surg 5:153-162, 1997.)

that the addition of recombinant BMP-2 to the autograft bone compensated for the inhibitory effect of ketorolac on bone formation.

KEY POINTS

✦ A trefoil-shaped canal increases the risk of lateral recess stenosis.
✦ When performing the physical examination, one must keep in mind that as we age, degenerative changes are common in the lumbar spine. Patients with stenosis may be asymptomatic.
✦ A CT/myelogram provides the best study for visualizing neural compression.

REFERENCES

1. Frishgrund J. Lumbar Degenerative Disorders of the Spine. Maine Review Course Lecture, 2003.
2. Herkowitz HN, Sidhu KS. Lumbar spine fusion in the treatment of degenerative conditions: Current indications and recommendations. J Am Acad Orthop Surg 3:123-135, 1995.
3. Amundsen T, Weber H, Lileas F, et al. Lumbar spinal stenosis: Clinical and radiographic features. Spine 20:1178-1186, 1995.
4. Bolender NF, Schonstrom NS, Spengler DM. Role of computed tomography and myelography in the diagnosis of central spinal stenosis. J Bone Joint Surg Am 67:240-246, 1985.
5. Spivak JM. Degenerative lumbar spinal stenosis [review]. J Bone Joint Surg Am 80:1053-1066, 1998.
6. Vad VB, Bhat AL, Lutz GE, et al. Transforaminal epidural steroid injections in lumbosacral radiculopathy. A prospective randomized study. Spine 27:11-16, 2002.
7. Cuckler JM, Bernini PA, Wiesel SW, et al. The use of epidural steroids in the treatment of lumbar radicular pain. A prospective, randomized, double-blind study. J Bone Joint Surg Am 67:63-66, 1985.
8. Dilke TF, Burry HC, Grahame R. Extradural corticosteroid injection in management of lumbar nerve root compression. Br Med J 2:635-637, 1973.
9. Holt EP Jr. The question of lumbar discography. J Bone Joint Surg Am 50:720-726, 1968.

10. Glassman SD, Rose SM, Dimar JR, et al. The effect of postoperative non-steroidal anti-inflammatory drug administration on spinal fusion. Spine 23: 834-838, 1998.
11. Herkowitz H. Surgical Options for "Discogenic" Low Back Pain. American Academy of Orthopaedic Surgeons Instructional Course, 2002.
12. Gill K, Blumenthal SL. Functional results after anterior lumbar fusion at L5-S1 in patients with normal and abnormal MRI scans. Spine 17:940-942, 1992.
13. Andersen T, Chrisensen FB, Laursen M, et al. Smoking as a predictor of negative outcome in lumbar spinal fusion. Spine 26:2623-2628, 2001.
14. American Academy of Orthopaedic Surgeons. Adult Spine Self-Assessment Examination. Orthopaedic Special Interest Examination, 2003.
15. Deguchi M, Rapoff AJ, Zdeblick TA. Posterolateral fusion for isthmic spondylolisthesis in adults: Analysis of fusion rate and clinical results. J Spinal Disord 11:459-464, 1998.
16. Glassman SD, Anagnost SC, Parker A, et al. The effect of cigarette smoking and smoking cessation on spinal fusion. Spine 25:2608-2615, 2000.
17. Snider RK, Krumwiede NK, Snider LJ, et al. Factors affecting lumbar spinal fusion. J Spinal Disord 12:107-114, 1999.
18. Martin GJ Jr, Boden SD, Titus L. Recombinant human bone morphogenetic protein-2 overcomes the inhibitory effect of ketorolac, a nonsteroidal anti-inflammatory drug (NSAID), on posterolateral lumbar intertransverse process spine fusion. Spine 24:2188-2193, 1999.

11 ▪ Diagnosis and Treatment of Sacroiliac Joint Pain: Sacrogenic Pain

Ralph F. Rashbaum

Because it is possible that more than one pain generator may coexist before the index spinal surgical procedure, Dr. David Polly, Professor of Orthopedic and Spine Surgery at the University of Minnesota, postulates that the incidence of failed back surgical syndrome can be measurably influenced. In those patients in whom it coexisted before surgery, it must be considered when formulating an initial surgical treatment plan.

PREVALENCE OF SACROILIAC JOINT PAIN

With the increasing number of fusions of the lumbar spine for axial low back pain caused by painful degeneration, spondyloarthropathy, instability, and deformity, studies[1-10] support the need to consider sacroiliac joint pain in the differential diagnosis of axial low back pain. Thirteen percent to 30% of patients with low back pain in general,[1-4] 29% to 43% of patients with postlumbar fusion surgery,[5-10] and 75% of patients 5 years after fusion had radiographic changes of the sacroiliac joint.[6] The incidence of sacroiliac joint degeneration was higher in patients who had fusion compared with patients who did not have fusion.[5]

In patients who have temporary resolution of their primary problem after surgery only to have axial lumbar pain return, it is essential to consider adjacent level degeneration (transitional syndrome) as a potential cause. The adjacent levels at risk of accelerated degeneration are the proximal spondylogenic segment and distally the sacrogenic segment.

Thus the physician will only be able to diagnose the cause and formulate an appropriate treatment plan to mitigate the resultant pain process if all the likely possibilities are understood. This chapter will help practitioners achieve the appropriate diagnosis and formulate a pathology-specific treatment plan. It is essential to make the correct diagnosis and find the primary pain generator based on an appropriate workup.

The sacroiliac joint has been called "the great impersonator." The presentation of pain radiating into and down the leg can lead to the primary diagnosis of a herniated disc. Radiation of pain to the groin and buttocks points to the hip joint as the source of pain. Both have specific radiographic findings and can easily be confirmed. The sacroiliac joint, however, often does not have significant changes on plain radiographs or CT scans.

The clinical presentation and a detailed examination will direct the physician to the sacroiliac joint as the source of pain. The following can help diagnose the appropriate site-specific cause of a patient's axial low back pain.

FIVE CAUSES OF AXIAL LOW BACK PAIN

The five causes of axial low back pain are diagnosed by interventional site-specific, fluoroscopically guided injections (i.e., "The" severe pain site for which the patient is seeking treatment).

1. Facetogenic: Spondylogenic facet arthrosis
   – Facet joint or medial branch block
2. Discogenic: Pain disc disruption
   – Anesthetic injections of the disc space
     • Functional ambulatory discography
3. Musculogenic: Chronic sprain/strain/postoperative myonecrosis
   – Trigger point
4. Sacrogenic: Sacroiliac disruption/dysfunction
   – Sacroiliac joint (lowermost portion of the joint)
5. Psychogenic: Psychogenic pain, symptom magnification (usually litigation involved)
   – Initial sequential differential pain study
   – Methohexital sodium (Brevital) pain study

SIGNS AND SYMPTOMS

■ Seated body posture leaning away from the painful side (Fig. 11-1, *A*).
■ Irregular gait with a shortened stride, an externally rotated foot, and partial forward flexion on the painful side.
■ Difficulty in standing from the seated posture (Fig. 11-1, *B*); the patient will stand on the painless side first and then shift his or her weight to balance on the painful side with an antalgic limp. The patient will have great difficulty getting into a recumbent posture; it is painful to get the pelvis level.
■ Fortin finger sign (Fig. 11-1, *C*).
■ Palm or knuckle sign (Fig. 11-1, *D*).
■ Pain drawings (Fig. 11-1, *E*).

Red Flag: All of the visual signs should raise the physician's awareness of the possibility that the sacroiliac joint is the patient's pain generator.

Fig. 11-1 A, The patient sits and rises with his body weight shifted to his nonpainful side. **B,** While transitioning to the standing position, the patient puts weight on the nonpainful side first and then shifts his weight to balance, which may be painful. **C,** One classic sign of sacroiliac joint pain is the Fortin finger sign, in which the patient uses one or two fingers to point directly over the painful sacroiliac joint. **D,** Patients with low back pain rather than sacroiliac joint pain tend to use the palm of their hand rather than a finger to indicate the painful area, located above the sacroiliac joint. **E,** Pain drawings may be helpful to differentiate the common origin of symptoms located in the low back region.

WORKUP

The examination is site specific to the sacroiliac joint.

Pain Provocation Tests

- Distraction (Fig. 11-2, *A*)
- Thigh thrust (Fig. 11-2, *B*)
- Flexion-abduction external rotation (FABER) test (Fig. 11-2, *C*)

Fig. 11-2   Several clinical evaluations used to evaluate a patient with possible sacroiliac joint pain. **A,** Distraction. **B,** Thigh thrust. **C,** FABER. (Courtesy of SI-BONE, San Jose, CA; with permission.)   *Continued*

Fig. 11-2, cont'd   D, Compression. **E,** Gaenslen maneuver. **F,** Stork sign. **G,** Resisted straight leg elevation. (Courtesy of SI-BONE, San Jose, CA; with permission.)

- Compression (Fig. 11-2, *D*)
- Gaenslen maneuver
  - Placement of the dorsum of the hand or rolled towel directly under the sacroiliac joint to increase leverage (Fig. 11-2, *E*)
- Stork sign (Fig. 11-2, *F*)
- Resisted straight leg elevation (Fig. 11-2, *G*)

Findings

- Tests proved to have a high degree of sensitivity and specificity for sacroiliac-derived pain
  - Distraction
    - ▸ Distraction has sensitivity values in the range of 85% to 91%, with 76% to 78% specificity.
  - Thigh thrust
    - ▸ The thigh thrust test has sensitivity values of 85% to 91%, with 76% to 78% specificity.
  - FABER
  - Compression
  - Gaenslen maneuver
- Most sensitive tests[11,12]
  - Distraction
    - ▸ Distraction has sensitivity values in the range of 85% to 91% with 76% to 78% specificity.
  - Thigh thrust
    - ▸ The thigh thrust test has sensitivity values of 85% to 91% and 76% to 78% specificity.

Blood Work (Nonspecific)

- Erythrocyte sedimentation rate
- C-reactive protein
- Complete blood cell count

Technetium Bone Scan

- Rarely positive, with the exceptions of spondyloarthropathies and infection

CT Scan

- Rarely helpful in achieving a diagnosis, but important in planning minimally invasive fusion of the sacroiliac joint

> **Red Flag:** There must be at least three positive results to provocation tests to proceed to the benchmark diagnostic test of fluoroscopically guided injection of the sacroiliac joint with anesthetics with or without steroids (diagnostic versus diagnostic/therapeutic).

Sacroiliac Joint Injection (Fig. 11-3)

- Nonresponsive, not the pain generator
- >75% pain reduction despite specific pain, positive

Fig. 11-3 Sacroiliac joint injection performed under fluoroscopic guidance.

- 50% to 75% pain reduction = equivocal
  - Repeat perhaps with CT guidance
  - Ask site-specific questions about pain relief (i.e., not a generalized pain score or residual pain).
- Pain specific to the location indicated by the Fortin finger test.
- Examine the patient 30 minutes after injection to determine whether provocation signs are gone.
- Sacroiliac injection technique
  - Inferiormost portion of the joint on AP projection with the C-arm inclined and rotated to maximize the joint space.
  - Limit the amount of contrast (Iohexol [Omnipaque 240]) injected (the joint will only accommodate up to 2.5 ml). It is most important to get the therapeutic medication into the joint.

> **Red Flag:** Use a 25-gauge spinal needle, because it will bend to accommodate entry into the joint.

TREATMENT/MANAGEMENT

The following measures should be considered when treating pain of sacroiliac origin

Conservative Treatment

- Physical therapy.
  - No data to support short- or long-term treatment
- Guarded weight-bearing with a walker or crutches.
- Chiropractic manipulation has temporary benefit in most patients.[13]
- Sacroiliac belt.
- NSAIDs.
  - No data to support short- or long-term treatment

- Analgesics
  - No data to support short- or long-term treatment
- Topicals
  - No data to support short- or long-term treatment

Invasive Treatment

- Prolotherapy
  - Not uniformly successful, but may reduce patients' symptoms to more tolerable levels.
  - Effect may be related to the neurolytic reaction to the noxious material that is used as the sclerosing agent.
- Medial branch rhizotomy
  - Usually L5, S1, S2, and S3 are targeted.
  - Clearly directed toward decreasing but not eliminating pain perception because not all of the dorsal innervation is addressed, whereas none of the ventral (abdominal) innervation is affected.[14]
  - Duration of benefits seems to be constrained by nerve regeneration between 6 and 12 months after rhizotomy.
- Neuromodulation
  - Standard epidural placement is not effective; no randomized controlled studies have been done.

Red Flag: Subcutaneous or field stimulation is investigational and is not covered by insurance.

- Fusion of the sacroiliac joint
  - Consider minimally invasive techniques, such as iFuse from SI-BONE (San Jose, CA) (Fig. 11-4, *A*).
    - ‣ This fusion approach deals directly with the mechanical cause of focal pain generation rather than modifying pain perception (Fig. 11-4, *B*).

Fig. 11-4   A, Implants used in minimally invasive fusion of the sacroiliac joint. **B,** A patient who underwent fusion of the sacroiliac joints bilaterally. (**A** Courtesy of SI-BONE; with permission.)

CONCLUSION

It is essential to consider each of the five causes of axial low back pain (facetogenic, discogenic, musculogenic, sacrogenic, and psychogenic) before a primary surgical plan is formulated. Failure to do so can lead to the creation of failed back surgery syndrome. The patient's history and presentation should be sufficient to elevate the physician's awareness of the possible causes of the patient's pain. The hands-on examination specifically directed toward the sacroiliac joint will add no more than 5 minutes; in every case it is time well spent. The definitive test after awareness has been raised is the injection of the sacroiliac joint under fluoroscopic guidance.

Confirmation is achieved when pain is reduced more than 75%. The right questions must be asked after injection. The pain of interest is site specific to the Fortin point test. In patients with previous spine surgery, residual neurogenic leg pain and any distant pain site should not be considered confirming.

Conservative therapy should be exhausted before surgical intervention. Failure to achieve an acceptable residual pain level in an attempt to preserve physical function should lead to the consideration of a mechanical solution to a mechanical problem: fusion of the sacroiliac joint by means of a minimally invasive technique.

KEY POINTS

✦ In patients who had temporary resolution of their primary problem after surgery only to have axial lumbar pain return, it is essential to consider adjacent level degeneration (transitional syndrome) as a potential cause.

✦ Visual cues exhibited by the patient, such as posture, gait, and the Fortin finger sign, should raise the physician's awareness of the possibility that the sacroiliac joint is the patient's pain generator.

✦ There must be at least three positive provocation tests to move on to the benchmark diagnostic test of fluoroscopically guided injection of the sacroiliac joint with anesthetics with or without steroids (diagnostic versus diagnostic/therapeutic).

✦ A 25-gauge spinal needle should be used when a sacroiliac joint injection is done because it will bend to accommodate entry into the joint.

✦ Subcutaneous or field stimulation is investigational and not covered by insurance.

REFERENCES

1. Maigne JY, Aivaliklis A, Pfefer F. Results of sacroiliac joint double block and value of sacroiliac pain provocation tests in 54 patients with low back pain. Spine 21:1889-1892, 1996.
2. Schwarzer AC, Aprill CN, Bogduk N. The sacroiliac joint in chronic low back pain. Spine 20:31-37, 1995.
3. Sembrano JN, Polly DW Jr. How often is low back pain not coming from the back? Spine 34:E27-E32, 2009.
4. Weksler N, Velan GJ, Semionov M, et al. The role of sacroiliac joint dysfunction in the genesis of low back pain: The obvious is not always right. Arch Orthop Trauma Surg 127:885-888, 2007.

5. DePalma MJ, Ketchum JM, Saullo TR. Etiology of chronic low back pain in patients having undergone lumbar fusion. Pain Med 12:732-739, 2011.

6. Ha KY, Lee JS, Kim KW. Degeneration of sacroiliac joint after instrumented lumbar or lumbosacral fusion: A prospective cohort study over five-year follow-up. Spine 33:1192-1198, 2008.

7. Ivanov AA, Kiapour A, Ebraheim NA, et al. Lumbar fusion leads to increases in angular motion and stress across sacroiliac joint: A finite element study. Spine 34:E162-E169, 2009.

8. Katz V, Schofferman J, Reynolds J. The sacroiliac joint: A potential cause of pain after lumbar fusion to the sacrum. J Spinal Disord Tech 16:96-99, 2003.

9. Liliang PC, Lu K, Liang CL, et al. Sacroiliac joint pain after lumbar and lumbosacral fusion: Findings using dual sacroiliac joint blocks. Pain Med 12:565-570, 2011.

10. Maigne JY, Planchon CA. Sacroiliac joint pain after lumbar fusion. A study with anesthetic blocks. Eur Spine J 14:654-658, 2005.

11. Laslett M, Aprill CN, McDonald B, et al. Diagnosis of sacroiliac joint pain: Validity of individual provocation tests and composites of tests. Man Ther 10:207-218, 2005.

12. Szadek KM, van der Wurff P, van Tulder MW, et al. Diagnostic validity of criteria for sacroiliac joint pain: A systematic review. J Pain 10:354-368, 2009.

13. Tullberg T, Blomberg S, Branth B, et al. Manipulation does not alter the position of the sacroiliac joint. A roentgen stereophotogrammetric analysis. Spine 23:1124-1128; discussion 1129, 1998.

14. Cohen SP, Hurley RW, Buckenmaier CC III, et al. Randomized placebo-controlled study evaluating lateral branch radiofrequency denervation for sacroiliac joint pain. Anesthesiology 109:279-288, 2008.

12 ▪ Spinal Cord Tumors

Rob D. Dickerman

Spinal tumors are generally classified into three categories based on anatomic location: extradural, intradural extramedullary, and intramedullary. Approximately 15% of primary central nervous system tumors are intramedullary. Metastatic tumors may be found in all three categories, but the majority are extradural.

CATEGORIES

1. Extradural: 55%; arise outside the spinal cord in vertebral bodies or epidural tissues.
2. Intradural extramedullary: 40%; arise in leptomeninges or roots. Most common are meningiomas and neurofibromas.
3. Intramedullary: 5%; arise within the spinal cord parenchyma. Typically invade gray matter and destroy spinal tracts.

EXTRADURAL SPINAL TUMORS

Most commonly, extradural spinal tumors are metastatic; they usually destroy the vertebral bodies or may cause epidural compression.

Metastatic Tumors

- Lymphoma: Secondary or metastatic lymphoma is the most common form of spinal lymphoma.
- Prostate: May be osteoblastic.

- Lung.
- Breast: May be osteoblastic.

Primary Spinal Tumors

- Chordoma: Clival and sacral regions.
- Vertebral hemangioma: May require preoperative embolization.
- Aneurysmal bone cyst.
- Neurofibromas: Characteristic "dumbbell-shaped" tumor on MRI.
- Osteoid osteoma: Night pains relieved with aspirin.
- Osteoblastoma: Night pains relieved with aspirin.

Intradural and/or Extradural Tumors

- Meningiomas: Up to 15% may be extradural.
- Neurofibromas (see p. 262).
- Angiolipoma.
- Chloroma: Focal collection of leukemic cells.

Spinal epidural metastases are the most common form of spinal tumor, occurring in up to 10% of cancer patients. Approximately 5% to 10% of malignancies present with the initial symptom of cord compression. The usual route of spread is hematogenous dissemination to the vertebral body, with erosion back through the pedicles and subsequent extension into the epidural space. Pain is the first symptom in 95% of patients. Pain may be focal, radicular, or referred and is exacerbated by movement, recumbency, a Valsalva maneuver, and straight-leg raising.

Diagnostic Studies

- Plain radiographs of the entire spine

Red Flag: Watch for pedicle erosion, "owl's eyes," or widening, indicative of pathologic compression fracture.

- Emergency MRI
  - MRI is the best diagnostic tool. Vertebral metastases are hypointense compared with normal bone marrow on T1-weighted images and hyperintense on T2-weighted images.
- Myelogram
  - Disadvantage: Invasive test.
  - Advantage: CSF is obtained.
- CT scan
  - Recommended for evaluation of bony erosion and anatomy.

Treatment/Management of Spinal Epidural Metastasis

- No treatment has been shown to prolong life.
- The goal of treatment is to control pain, preserve spinal stability, and maintain sphincter control as well as the ability to ambulate.
- Primary surgical options:
  - Surgery only
  - Surgery and postoperative radiation
  - Radiation only
- The most important factor affecting prognosis, regardless of treatment modality, is the patient's ability to walk at the time therapy is initiated. Loss of sphincter control is a poor prognosticator and is often irreversible.[1]

INTRADURAL EXTRAMEDULLARY

Most commonly, intradural extramedullary tumors are meningiomas and fibromas.

Meningiomas

- Arise from arachnoid cap cells.
- 99% are benign.
- May have significant edema.
- Dural tail may light up on MRI.

- Prognosis depends on the degree of resection.
- May require dural graft.

Neurofibroma (not encapsulated)

- Localized, diffuse, or plexiform.
- Classic dumbbell shape.
- Associated with neurofibromatosis.[1]
- Tumor is within nerve fibers.
- Surgery is reserved for large, painful tumors. The risk-to-benefit ratio of surgical nerve resection must be considered; 10% of these tumors may undergo malignant transformation.

Schwannoma (Encapsulated) Tumor of Nerve Sheath

- Use nerve stimulator to identify nerve fascicles intraoperatively.

Lipoma (see below)

- Metastatic
- Occurrence: Approximately 4%

Diagnostic Studies

- MRI is the study of choice.
- Meningiomas: Homogenous enhancement and usually demonstrate a classic "dural tail."
- Neurofibromas show a typical dumbbell shape on MRI.
- Lipomas typically occur in the region of the conus but may be throughout the spine. High signal intensity on T2-weighted MRI.

Treatment/Management

- For meningiomas, the goal is complete resection. The recurrence rate with complete resection is approximately 7%. (The recurrence rate is dependent on the degree of resection.) Stereotactic radiation is recommended in subtotal resection cases.

- CyberKnife and linear accelerator both offer certain advantages, depending on tumor type, size, and location.
- Neurofibromas may be idiopathic or associated with neurofibromatosis. Gross total resection is the goal. The obvious risk-to-benefit consideration of sacrificing the nerve must be discussed with the patient before surgery. The recurrence rate is high.
- A lipoma may be intradural and significantly entangled within the nerve roots or conus. Microdissection is essential with monitoring, and direct nerve stimulation is helpful.

INTRAMEDULLARY

Intrinsic central nervous system (CNS) tumor. Use "rule of 30%": 30% astrocytoma, 30% ependymoma, and 30% miscellaneous.

Astrocytoma[2,3]

- 30%: The most common intramedullary spinal cord tumor outside the filum terminale.
- Most commonly occurs in the thoracic spine.
- Peak ages are the third to sixth decades of life.
- 40% may be cystic.

Ependymoma[3,4]

- 30%: Most common glioma of the lower spinal cord, conus; >50% occur in the filum.
- Cystic degeneration in >40% of cases.
- Peak ages are the third to fifth decades of life.
- Myxopapillary ependymoma has no anaplasia; characteristically papillary with microcytic vacuoles.
- Surgical removal requires coagulating and dividing the filum just above or below the lesion. The filum is first cut above the lesion to prevent cephalad retraction of the lesion. Under the microscope, the filum has a distinctively whiter appearance than nerve roots and a characteristic squiggly vessel on the surface of the filum. Intra-

operative monitoring with direct stimulation of roots and anal sphincter monitoring are required.

Less Common Intramedullary Tumors

- Hemangioblastoma[5]
  - Associated with von Hippel-Lindau disease; highly vascular: requires meticulous dissection and identification of feeding arteries.

Red Flag: Must attack circumferentially—do not go inside-outside!

  - May have syrinx-cyst; use the cyst as an operative approach to the tumor.
  - Indocyanine green videoangiography provides real-time intraoperative visualization of tumor vasculature.[6]
- Lipoma[7]
  - May occur with spinal dysraphism.
  - Epidural lipomatosis associated with Cushing's disease.
  - Peak ages are the second to fifth decades of life.
  - Cervicothoracic region is the most common site.
  - Symptoms include ascending monoparesis or paraparesis.
  - Sphincter disturbance is common in lower lesions.
- Teratoma
- Epidermoid
  - Can occur as a result of lumbar puncture.
- Dermoid
- Glioblastoma
- Metastastic
  - Less than 2% of metastatic tumors of the spine
- Inflammatory masses[8,9]
  - May mimic symptoms of intrinsic tumor.
- Sarcoidosis

Presentation

- Pain is the most common complaint; characteristic pain during recumbency (nocturnal pain) is classic with spinal cord tumors.[10]
- May involve a syrinx with dysesthesias, nonradicular.
- Weakness is the second most common complaint.
- Long-tract findings include clumsiness, ataxia.
- Fasciculations, muscle twitches, atrophy occur.
- Syringomyelic syndrome is classic for intramedullary tumor; involves dissociated sensory loss (decreased pain and temperature with preserved light touch).
- Urinary sphincter disturbances include retention or incontinence and impotence. Anal sphincter disturbances are not as common.
- Symptoms may be present for up to 2 years before diagnosis because of the slow growth rate of this type of tumor.

Diagnostic Studies

- Plain radiographs
  - Demonstrate vertebral body destruction; enlarged foramen or increases in interpedicular distance suggest extradural spinal tumor.
  - Preoperative radiographic marking by radiologist can reduce unnecessary surgical exposure intraoperatively.
- Myelogram
  - Demonstrates fusiform widening for intramedullary tumors versus an hourglass deformity with incomplete block in extradural tumors or paintbrush effect with complete block.
  - Intradural extramedullary tumors produce the meniscus sign, a capping effect with a sharp cutoff.
- CT scans
  - Some intramedullary tumors are enhanced with IV contrast.
- MRI
  - Best diagnostic tool.

- Virtually all intramedullary tumors will show cord expansion, widening, thickening.[9]
- Scanning entire craniospinal axis should be considered to rule out a dropped CNS tumor.
- Spinal angiography
  - Typically indicated for hemangioblastomas.[5]

Differential Diagnosis

- Vascular lesions: AVM.
- Demyelinating disease: Multiple sclerosis.
- Inflammatory myelitis.
- Paraneoplastic myelopathy.
- Diseases of vertebral body: Giant cell tumors, Paget's disease.

Prognosis

- Results are most dependent on the patient's preoperative functional status.[11]
- Recurrence depends on the degree of extirpation and on the growth pattern of the specific tumor.[3]
- Ependymoma: Total resection improves functional outcome, and myxopapillary ependymomas fare better than the classic type.[3]
- Astrocytoma: Radical resection rarely possible. Long-term outcomes worse than ependymomas. There is a 50% recurrence rate in 4-5 years. For high-grade lesions, radiation treatment is recommended postoperatively.[2,12,13]

KEY POINTS

+ Three primary determinants of outcome are preoperative neurofunctional status, histology, and the degree of surgical resection.[11]
+ A syrinx is either tumor, posttraumatic, postinfectious, or Chiari malformation (abnormal CSF flow).
+ 99% of intrinsic spinal cord tumors will show cord expansion on MRI.[9]

+ Astrocytomas have a difficult cleavage plane; this requires spinal cord monitoring; both SSEP and transcortical motor evoked potentials are recommended. For high-grade tumors, the surgeon should plan intraoperatively to "do no harm"; aggressive resection may be too high risk.[4]

+ Wide tumors on MRI are generally worse because the corticospinal tracts are pushed anteriorly and laterally.

+ Intramedullary surgery requires meticulous control of bleeding, not only for visualization but also because blood is an irritant to the CNS, which can cause postoperative fevers and increase the risk for infection.

+ Some surgeons advocate taking 40 mg of propranolol (for the surgeon) before spinal cord tumor surgery to increase the steadiness of their hands.

+ The obvious goal of intramedullary surgery is gross total resection; however, the specific pathology dictates the degree of surgical aggressiveness.[11]

+ A midline myelotomy at the thinnest portion of the cord should always be used unless the tumor presents dorsally.[14]

+ Preoperative radiographic skin marking by a radiologist can reduce unnecessary surgical exposure intraoperatively.

+ Intraoperative ultrasonography is helpful in localizing the tumor before durotomy.[15]

+ Cavitron ultrasonic surgical aspirator (CUSA) is helpful in debulking certain tumors.[16]

+ The surgeon must always be extremely alert while dissecting ventral to the anterior spinal artery.

+ Corticospinal tracts may be splayed anteriorly and laterally.

+ When performing diagnostic studies for extradural tumors, watch for pedicle erosion, "owl's eyes," or widening, indicative of pathologic compression fracture.

+ When treating hemangioblastomas, attack them circumferentially—do not go inside-outside.

REFERENCES

1. Schiff D, O'Neill BP, Suman VJ. Spinal epidural metastasis as the initial manifestation of malignancy: Clinical features and diagnostic approach. Neurology 49:452-456, 1997.
2. Jallo GI, Danish S, Velasquez L, et al. Intramedullary low-grade astrocytomas: Long-term outcome following radical surgery. J Neurooncol 53:61-66, 2001.
3. Jallo GI, Kothbauer KF, Epstein FJ. Intrinsic spinal cord tumor resection. Neurosurgery 49:1124-1128, 2001.
4. Quinones-Hinojosa A, Lyon R, Zada G, et al. Changes in transcranial motor evoked potentials during intramedullary spinal cord tumor resection correlate with postoperative motor function. Neurosurgery 56:982-993, 2005.
5. Pluta RM, Iuliano B, DeVroom HL, et al. Comparison of anterior and posterior surgical approaches in the treatment of ventral spinal hemangioblastomas in patients with von Hippel-Lindau disease. J Neurosurg 98:117-124, 2003.
6. Hao S, Di L, Ma G, et al. Application of intraoperative indocyanine green videoangiography for resection of spinal cord hemagioblastoma: Advantages and limitations. J Clin Neurosci 20:1269-1275, 2013.
7. Bhatoe HS, Singh P, Chaturvedi A, et al. Nondysraphic intramedullary spinal cord lipomas: A review. Neurosurg Focus 18, 2005.
8. Dickerman RD, Colle K, Mittler MA. Intramedullary inflammatory mass dorsal to the Klippel-Feil deformity: Error in development or response to an abnormal motion segment? Spinal Cord 42:720-722, 2004.
9. Lee M, Epstein FJ, Rezai AR, et al. Nonneoplastic intramedullary spinal cord lesions mimicking tumors. Neurosurgery 43:788-794, 1998.
10. Houten JK, Cooper PR. Spinal cord astrocytomas: Presentation, management and outcome. J Neurooncol 47:219-224, 2000.
11. Raco A, Esposito V, Lenzi J, et al. Long-term follow-up of intramedullary spinal cord tumors: A series of 202 cases. Neurosurgery 56:972-981, 2005.
12. Klimo P, Thompson CJ, Kestle JR, et al. A meta-analysis of surgery versus conventional radiotherapy for the treatment of metastatic spinal epidural disease. Neurooncology 7:64-76, 2005.
13. Zorlu F, Ozyigit G, Gurkaynak M, et al. Postoperative radiotherapy results in primary spinal cord astrocytomas. Radiother Oncol 74:45-48, 2005.
14. McCormick PC, Stein BM. Intramedullary tumors in adults. Neurosurg Clin North Am 1:609-630, 1990.
15. Epstein FJ, Farmer JP, Schneider SJ. Intraoperative ultrasonography: An important surgical adjunct for intramedullary tumors. J Neurosurg 74:729-733, 1991.
16. Epstein F. The Cavitron ultrasonic aspirator in tumor surgery. Clin Neurosurg 31:497-505, 1983.

Appendix

GLOSSARY

complete injury   Absence of sensory and motor function in the lowest sacral segment.

decompensation   C7 plumb line in relation to pelvis.

dermatome   Area of the skin innervated by the sensory axons within each segmental nerve (root).

incomplete injury   If partial preservation of sensory and/or motor functions is found below the neurologic level *and* includes the lowest sacral segment, the injury is defined as incomplete. Sacral sensation includes sensation at the anal mucocutaneous junction as well as deep anal sensation. The test of motor function is the presence of voluntary contraction of the external anal sphincter upon digital examination.

Lenke stable vertebra   The most proximal vertebra that is classified as an A or B (lumbar modifier). When the neutral vertebra and the stable vertebra do not correspond, the data suggest that fusion to the stable vertebra will give the most reliable and satisfactory long-term result.

myotome   Collection of muscle fibers innervated by the motor axons within each segmental nerve (root).

Nash-Moe   System used for determining pedicle rotation. The vertebral body is divided into six segments and grades from 0 to 4 are assigned, depending on the location of the pedicle within segments. Because the pedicle on the concave side disappears early in rotation, pedicle on convex side, easily visible through wide range of rotation, is used as standard 5.

neurologic level, sensory level, motor level   *Neurologic level* refers to the caudalmost segment of the spinal cord with normal sensory and motor function on both sides of the body. In fact, the segments at which normal function is found often differ by side of body and in terms of sensory versus motor testing. Thus up to four different segments may be identified in determining the neurologic level: R-sensory, L-sensory, R-motor, L-motor. In cases such as this, it is strongly recommended that each of these segments be separately recorded and that a single "level" not be used, since this can be misleading in such cases. When the term *sensory level* is used, it refers to the caudalmost segment of the spinal cord with normal sensory function on both sides of the body; the *motor level* is similarly defined with respect to motor function. These "levels" are determined by neurologic examination of (1) a key sensory point within each of 28 dermatomes on the right and 28 dermatomes on the left side of the body, and (2) a key muscle within each of 10 myotomes on the right and 10 myotomes on the left side of the body.

neutral vertebra   The neutral vertebra is determined by the criteria established by Nash and Moe. It can be established when both pedicles are symmetrical on the posteroanterior radiograph and spinous process is seen equidistant between the pedicles.

odontoid fracture   Cervical spine fracture that involves the tip, junction, and body. Type II is more commonly associated with malunion. Congenital stenosis (<0.8 on CT) ratio of canal/body is defined by the parathesis.

parallel disc   Refers to the endplates of two adjacent vertebral bodies that have no wedge. Wedging of the endplates is usually seen. This disc is usually superior to the stable vertebral body.

paraplegia   Impairment or loss of motor and/or sensory function in the thoracic, lumbar, or sacral (but not cervical) segments of the spinal cord, resulting from damage of neural elements within the spinal canal. In paraplegia arm functioning is spared, but, depending on the level of injury, the trunk, legs, and pelvic organs may be involved.

push-prone radiograph   In addition to supine AP radiographs, this is the other helpful predictor of spontaneous lumbar curve correction. The patient is placed prone on the radiograph table while manual pressure is applied to the apex of the thoracic curve at the same time the pelvis and shoulders are stabilized. An AP radiograph is taken of the entire spine. The residual lumbar curve measurement represents the amount of spontaneous lumbar curve correction that would be expected with a selective thoracic instrumented fusion. Correction of the thoracic curve should not exceed the spontaneous correction of the lumbar curve on the push-prone radiograph to avoid decompensation of the lumbar curve.

reverse rotation   Spinous processes of the thoracic and lumbar spine are in opposite directions. Reverse rotation is usually seen in 1A, 1B classification. In instrumentation in the reverse rotation, the instrumentation should not end at the parallel disc, because it is part of the lumbar curve, and the reverse rotation tips the surgeon to that. As opposed to nonreverse rotation, the parallel disc should be included in the instrumentation.

sagittal plane   Sagittal sacral line used to prevent junctional kyphosis in posterior spinal fusion (PSF). If the patient is kyphotic, a more stable bisected end vertebra is required, whereas in a scoliotic patient without sagittal deformity, the end vertebrae just need to be touching.

sagittal stable vertebra   Line drawn vertically from posterior sacral vertebral body. The last vertebra touched by the line is the stable vertebra and it is safe to stop instrumentation at this point.

sensory scores, motor scores   Numerical summary scores that reflect the degree of neurologic impairment associated with the spinal cord injury (SCI).

skeletal level   The level at which, by radiographic examination, the greatest vertebral damage is found.

stable vertebra   The center sacral vertical line is extended in a cephalad direction as a perpendicular line from a line horizontally connecting superior portion of iliac crests, and the cephaladmost lumbar or thoracic vertebra most closely bisected by the line is considered the stable vertebra. When limb-length discrepancy is present, the pelvis should be leveled with an appropriate lift under the short limb. The central vertical line must always be based on a horizontal pelvis.

tetraplegia (preferred to "quadriplegia")   Impairment or loss of motor and/or sensory function in the cervical segments of the spinal cord as a result of damage of neural elements within the spinal canal. Tetraplegia results in impairment of function in the arms as well as in the trunk, legs, and pelvic organs. It does not include brachial plexus lesions or injury to peripheral nerves outside the neural canal.

trunk shift   Position of the ribcage in relationship to the pelvis.

zone of partial preservation (ZPP)   Dermatomes and myotomes caudal to the neurologic level that remain partially innervated. When some impaired sensory and/or motor function is found below the lowest normal segment, the exact number of segments so affected should be recorded for both sides as the ZPP. The term is used only with complete injuries.

ABBREVIATIONS

AADI	Anterior atlantodens interval
ACDF	Anterior cervical disc fusion
ALIF	Anterior lumbar interbody fusion
amp	Ampule
aPTT	Activated partial thromboplastin time
ATR	Angle of trunk rotation
AVR	Apical vertebral rotation
AVT	Apical vertebral translation
bid	Twice per day
BMP	Bone morphogenetic protein
BP	Blood pressure
CHF	Congestive heart failure
COX	Cyclooxygenase
CSVL	Center sacral vertical line
CTLSO	Cervicothoracolumbosacral orthosis
CUSA	Cavitron ultrasonic surgical aspirator
CVA	Cerebrovascular accident
D/C	Discontinue
DDD	Degenerative disc disease
DTR	Deep tendon reflex
DVT	Deep vein thrombosis
EMG	Electromyograph; electromyogram
FABER	Flexion-abduction external rotation
GCS	Glasgow Coma Scale
IDET	Internal disc electrotherapy
IM	Intramuscularly
INR	International Normalized Ratio for prothrombin activity
IPPB	Intermittent positive pressure breathing
IS	Intercostal space
IV	Intravenously
LE	Lower extremities
LOC	Loss of consciousness

MI	Myocardial infarction
MSPQ	Modified Somatic Perceptions Questionnaire
NSAIDs	Nonsteroidal antiinflammatory drugs
O₂	Oxygen
OPLL	Ossification of the posterior longitudinal ligament
PADI	Posterior atlantodens interval
PCA	Patient-controlled analgesia
PE	Pulmonary embolism
PLIF	Posterior lumbar interbody fusion
PO	By mouth; orally
POD	Postoperative day
PR	By rectum
PSF	Posterior spinal fusion
PSIS	Posterior superior iliac spine
PT	Prothrombin time
PTT	Partial thromboplastin time
qd	Every day
q hr	Every hour
qid	Four times per day
RhA	Rheumatoid arthritis
RVAD	Rib-vertebral angle difference
SAC	Subaxial canal
SCD	Sequential compression device
SCI	Spinal cord injury
SEP	Somatosensory evoked potential
SL	Sublingually
SMO	Superior migration of the odontoid
SPECT	Single-photon emission computed tomography
SQ	Subcutaneously
SSEP	Spinal somatosensory evoked potential
tab	Tablet
TEDS	Antiembolism stockings
TFESIs	Transforaminal epidural steroid injections

tid	Three times per day
TKO	To keep open
TLIF	Transforaminal lumbar interbody fusion
TLSO	Thoracolumbosacral orthosis
UE	Upper extremities
VAS	Visual Analog Scale
VCF	Vertebral compression fractures
ZDI	Zung Depression Index

Index